Healthy Meal Prep Cookbook

1800 Days of Easy & Vibrant Recipes, Convenient & Quicky Make Ahead Homemade Food List | Take Nutrition and Health with You | No Waste

Kercival Wterlly

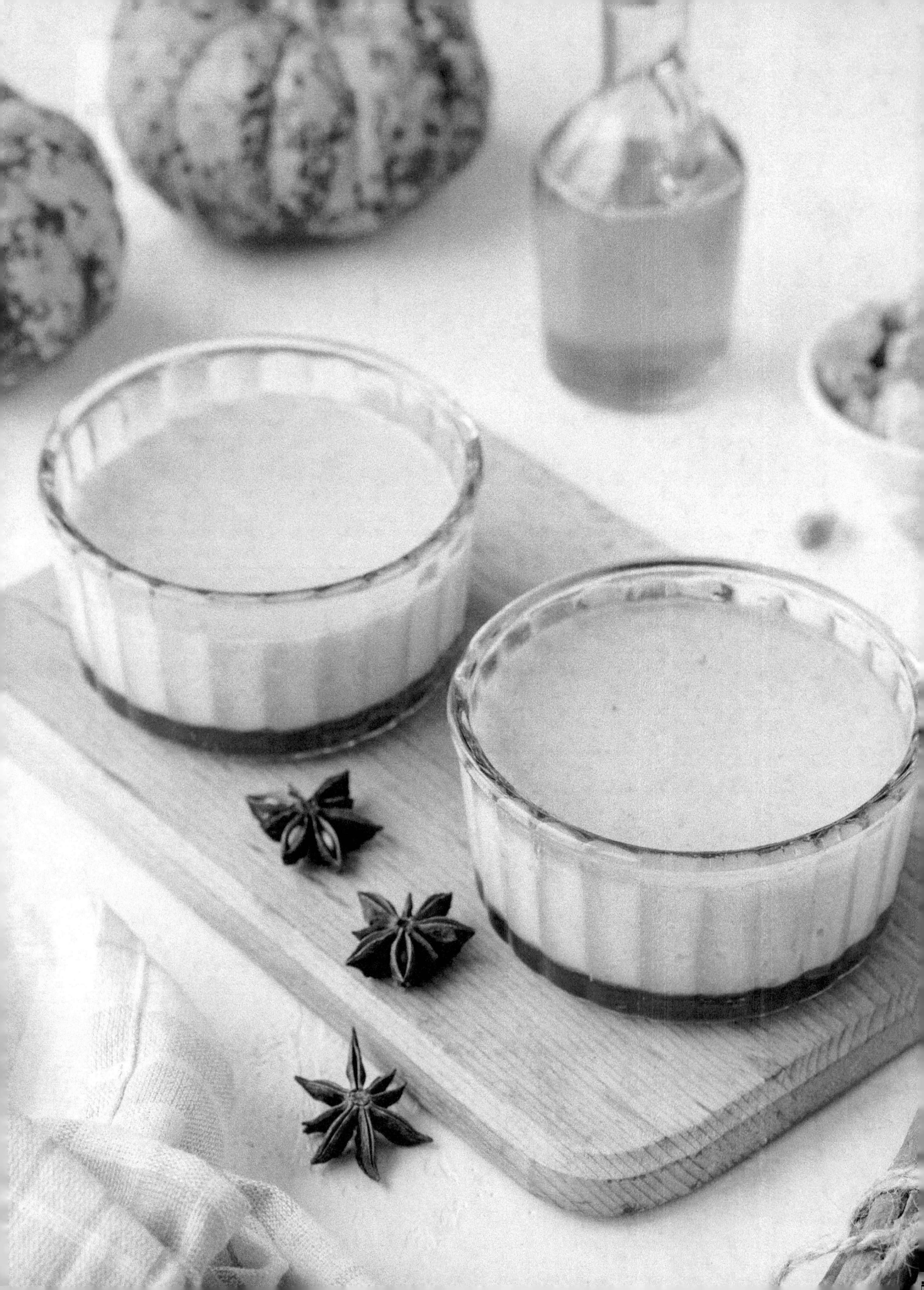

Table of Contents

INTRODUCTION

What is Meal Prep?

Meal prep, short for meal preparation, is a practice of planning and preparing meals in advance, typically for a week, to save time and promote healthier eating habits. It involves cooking and assembling ingredients ahead of time, so that when it's time to eat, the majority of the work is already done. This concept has gained significant popularity in recent years, driven by the desire for convenience, healthier eating, and efficient time management.

The process of meal prep generally includes several key steps:

- Planning: The first step in meal prep is to plan your meals for the week. This involves deciding what recipes you'll make, considering nutritional balance, variety, and portion control.

- Grocery Shopping: Once you have a meal plan, you can create a shopping list for the ingredients you need. This step helps in avoiding last-minute trips to the grocery store and impulse purchases.

- Preparation: With all the ingredients on hand, the next step is to prepare the components of your meals. This can include washing and chopping vegetables, marinating proteins, and cooking grains or legumes.

- Cooking: The actual cooking of the meals takes place during this step. It can involve baking, roasting, grilling, or any other cooking method that suits the recipes you've chosen.

- Portioning: After the meals are cooked, they are portioned into individual servings. This step is crucial for controlling calorie intake and ensuring balanced nutrition.

- Storage: Once portioned, the meals are stored in containers. Proper storage helps maintain freshness and prevents spoilage. It also makes it easy to grab a pre-prepared meal when needed.

- Reheating (if necessary): Some meals may need to be reheated before

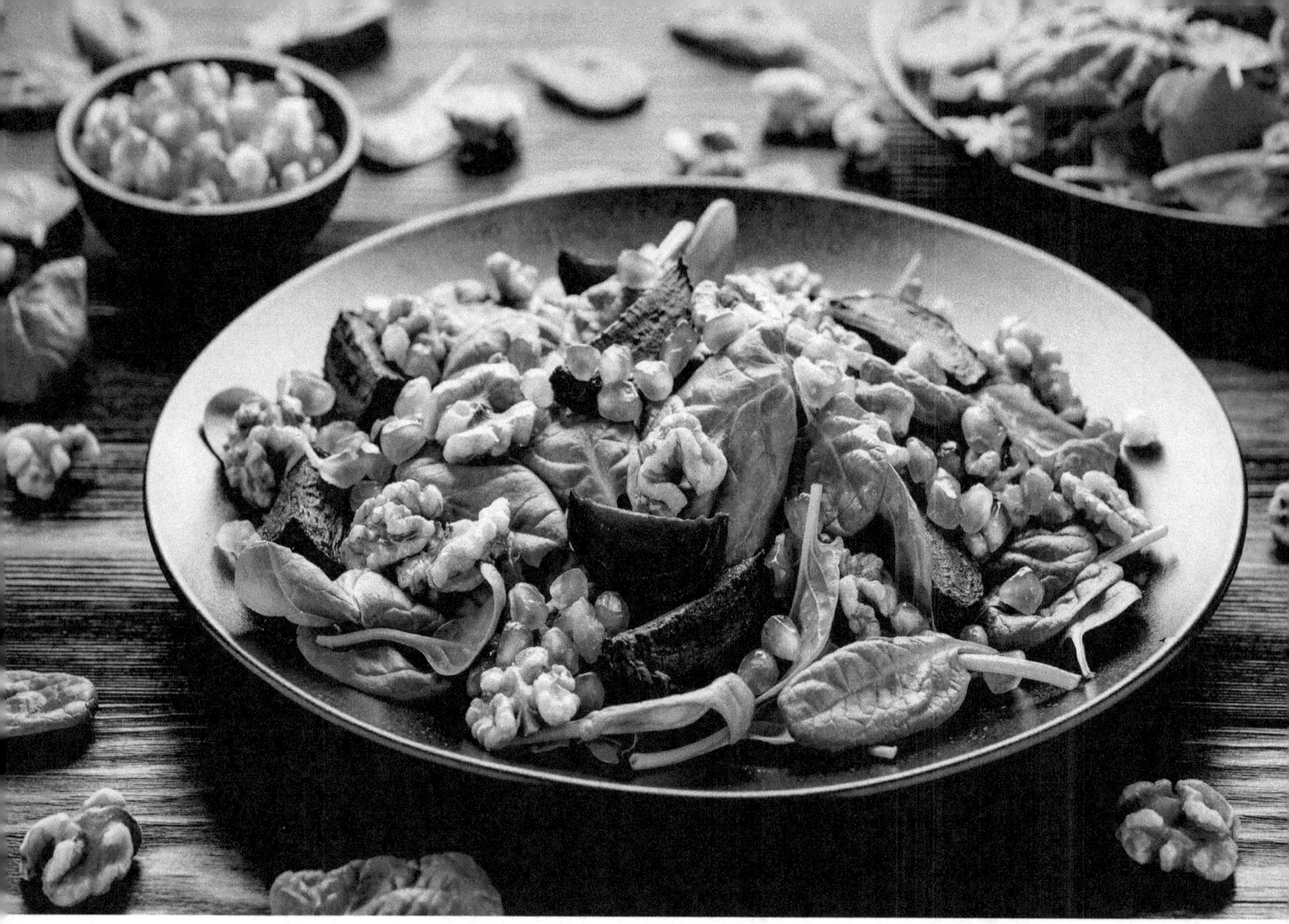

consumption. Having a plan for reheating ensures that the meals are still tasty and satisfying.

- Meal prep offers numerous benefits, making it a popular approach for those with busy lifestyles or specific health goals:

- Time Savings: By dedicating a few hours to meal prep on a designated day, individuals can save a significant amount of time during the week. This is especially beneficial for those with hectic schedules.

- Consistent Nutrition: Planning meals in advance allows for better control over nutritional content. It facilitates the creation of balanced meals with the right mix of macronutrients and micronutrients.

- Cost-Effective: Buying ingredients in bulk and planning meals strategically can help reduce food waste and overall grocery expenses.

- Healthier Choices: When healthy meals are readily available, individuals are less likely to resort to fast food or unhealthy snacks. This can contribute to weight management and overall well-being.

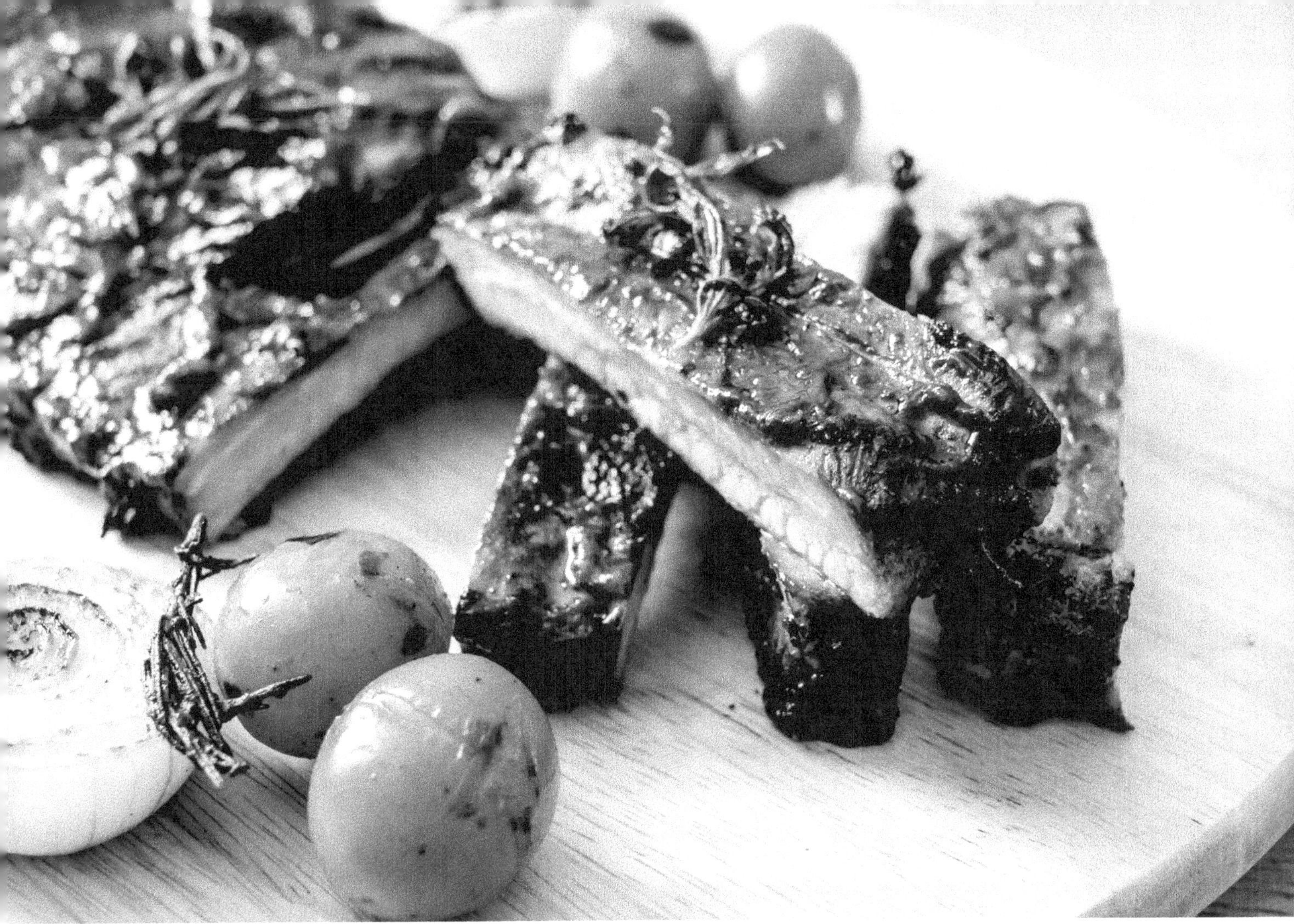

- Portion Control: Pre-portioned meals make it easier to control portion sizes, aiding in weight management and preventing overeating.
- Reduced Stress: Knowing that meals are already prepared can alleviate the stress of deciding what to eat each day and the time-consuming process of cooking from scratch.

In the context of a Healthy Meal Prep Cookbook, the recipes included would focus on nutrient-dense ingredients, lean proteins, whole grains, and a variety of fruits and vegetables. The cookbook would likely provide a diverse range of recipes to keep meals interesting and enjoyable, catering to different dietary preferences and restrictions.

In essence, meal prep is a practical and effective approach to eating well, saving time, and aligning with health and wellness goals. The Healthy Meal Prep Cookbook serves as a valuable resource, guiding individuals through the process of planning, preparing, and enjoying nutritious meals that contribute to a healthier and more balanced lifestyle.

Benefits of Meal Prep

Meal prepping has gained immense popularity in recent years, and for good reason. It is not just a trend but a lifestyle choice that brings along a plethora of benefits. Whether you are a busy professional, a fitness enthusiast, or someone looking to maintain a healthier lifestyle, incorporating meal prep into your routine can be a game-changer. Let's delve into the various advantages of meal prep that go beyond just saving time.

Time Efficiency:

One of the most apparent benefits of meal prep is the time saved. In our fast-paced lives, finding time to cook healthy meals every day can be challenging. Meal prepping allows you to dedicate a specific block of time, usually on the weekends, to prepare and portion out your meals for the entire week. This means less time spent in the kitchen on busy weekdays and more time for other priorities.

Consistent Portion Control:

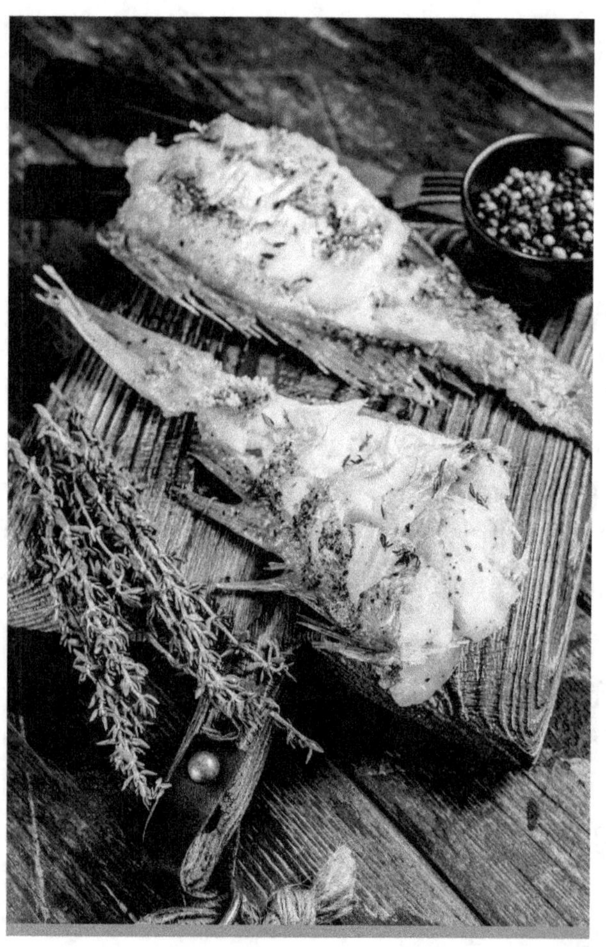

Meal prepping promotes portion control, a key factor in maintaining a healthy diet. When you prepare your meals in advance, you have better control over the quantity of each ingredient, helping you avoid overeating. This is particularly crucial for those looking to manage or lose weight as it eliminates the temptation to indulge in oversized portions.

Nutrient-Rich Choices:

When you plan your meals ahead of time, you can focus on creating a well-balanced and nutrient-dense menu. This ensures that your body receives the essential vitamins, minerals, and macronutrients it needs for optimal functioning. You can incorporate a variety of colorful fruits, vegetables, lean proteins, and whole grains into your meals, contributing to a well-rounded and wholesome diet.

Financial Savings:

Meal prepping can also lead to significant financial savings. Buying ingredients in bulk and preparing meals at home is often more cost-effective than dining out or buying pre-packaged convenience foods regularly. Additionally, by having a plan and a prepared shopping list, you are less likely to make impulse purchases, reducing overall food expenses.

Reduces Stress:

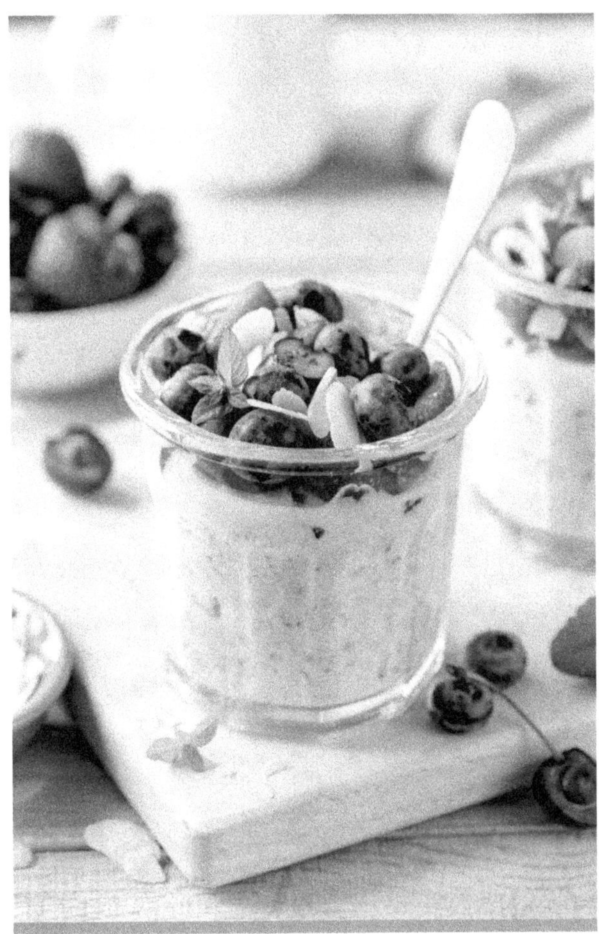

The daily decision of what to cook can be a source of stress for many individuals. Meal prepping eliminates this daily dilemma as your meals are already planned and prepared. This can be especially beneficial for those with busy schedules, reducing the mental load and providing a sense of order and control over your nutrition.

Healthier Food Choices:

When you have nutritious meals readily available, you are less likely to opt for unhealthy, convenient alternatives. Having a fridge stocked with prepped meals ensures that you always have a healthy option on hand, making it easier to resist the temptation of fast food or processed snacks.

Customization and Variety:

Meal prepping doesn't mean eating the same meal every day. In fact, it allows for creativity and variety in your diet. You can experiment with different recipes, flavors, and cuisines, ensuring that your meals remain interesting and satisfying. This variety also helps prevent boredom and promotes a more sustainable approach to healthy eating.

In conclusion, the benefits of meal prep extend far beyond the convenience of having meals ready in advance. It is a powerful tool for promoting overall health

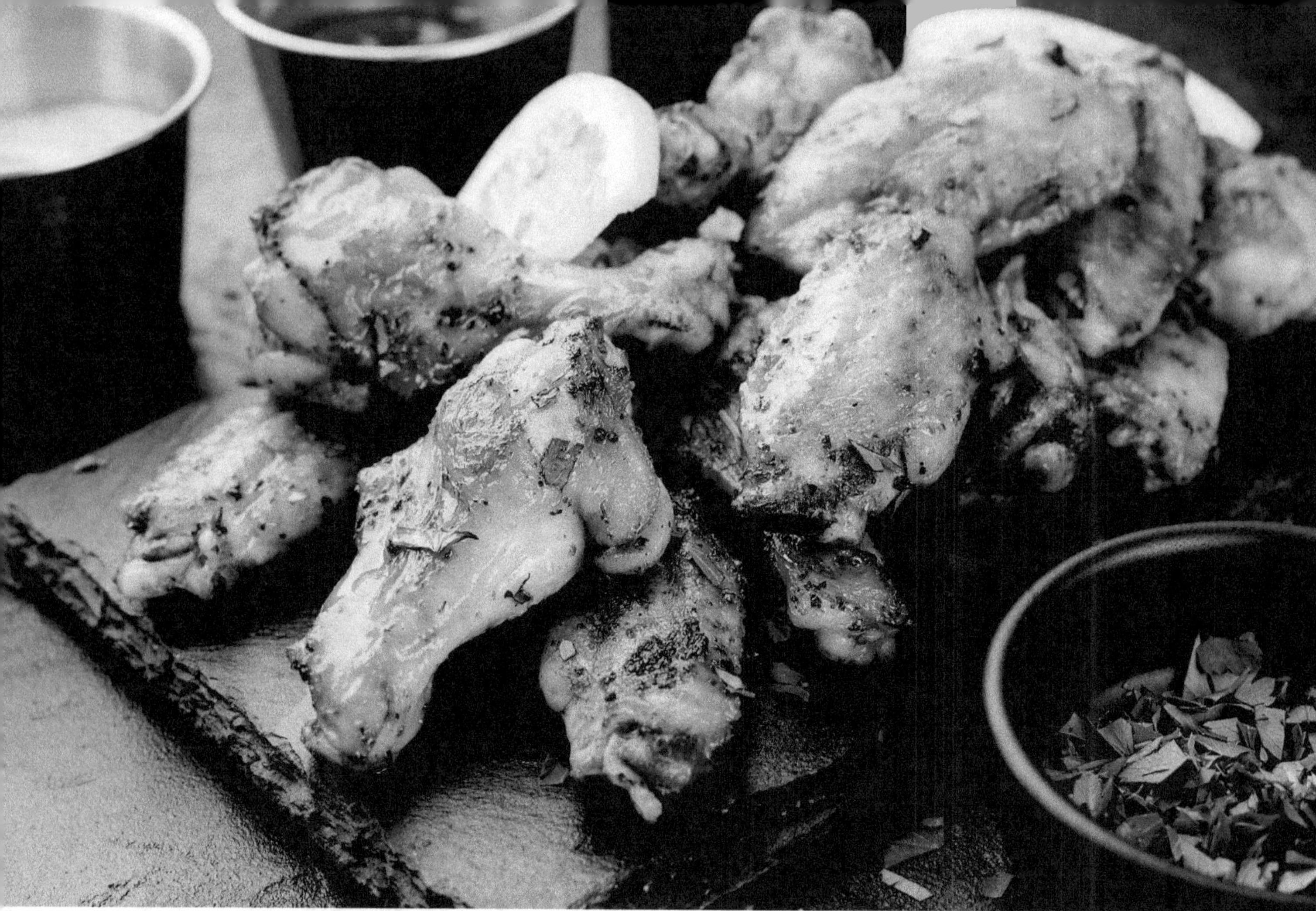

and well-being by saving time, supporting portion control, ensuring a nutrient-rich diet, and contributing to financial savings. Making meal prep a consistent part of your routine can lead to positive and lasting changes in your lifestyle.

What You'll Need for Big-Batch Cooking?

Big-batch cooking is an excellent strategy for those who want to maintain a healthy and convenient lifestyle. It involves preparing large quantities of food at once, allowing you to have ready-made meals throughout the week. To embark on successful big-batch cooking for a Healthy Meal Prep Cookbook, you'll need the right ingredients, equipment, and a well-thought-out plan.

Quality Ingredients:

The foundation of any healthy meal is the quality of its ingredients. When planning for big-batch cooking, prioritize fresh, whole foods. Opt for a variety of vegetables, lean proteins, whole grains, and legumes. Incorporate a rainbow of colors in your vegetables to ensure a diverse range of nutrients. Selecting high-quality ingredients not only enhances the nutritional profile of your meals but also contributes to better taste and overall satisfaction.

Lean Proteins:

Proteins are essential for muscle repair and overall body function. Include lean protein sources like skinless poultry, lean beef, fish, tofu, and legumes. These proteins will not only provide essential amino acids but also keep your meals filling and satisfying.

Whole Grains:

Whole grains are rich in fiber and complex carbohydrates, providing sustained energy and promoting digestive health. Quinoa, brown rice, bulgur, and oats are excellent choices for big-batch cooking. They serve as a base for various dishes and can be easily reheated without compromising texture or taste.

Assorted Vegetables:

Load up on a variety of vegetables to ensure a diverse nutrient intake. Broccoli, spinach, bell peppers, carrots, and tomatoes are versatile options that can be incorporated into different recipes. Vegetables not only add flavor and texture but also contribute essential vitamins and minerals.

Healthy Fats:

Incorporate sources of healthy fats to enhance the flavor and nutritional content of your meals. Avocado, olive oil, nuts, and seeds are excellent choices. These fats play a crucial role in nutrient absorption and provide a sense of satiety.

Herbs and Spices:

Seasonings are the secret to turning simple ingredients into flavorful meals. Stock up on a variety of herbs and spices to add depth and complexity to your dishes without relying on excessive salt or sugar. Fresh herbs like basil, cilantro, and thyme, along with spices such as cumin, turmeric, and paprika, can transform your big-batch meals into culinary delights.

Storage Containers:

Invest in a variety of high-quality storage containers to keep your big-batch meals fresh. Choose containers that are microwave-safe and have airtight seals to maintain the integrity of your dishes. Divided containers are particularly useful for keeping different components of your meals separate until you're ready to eat.

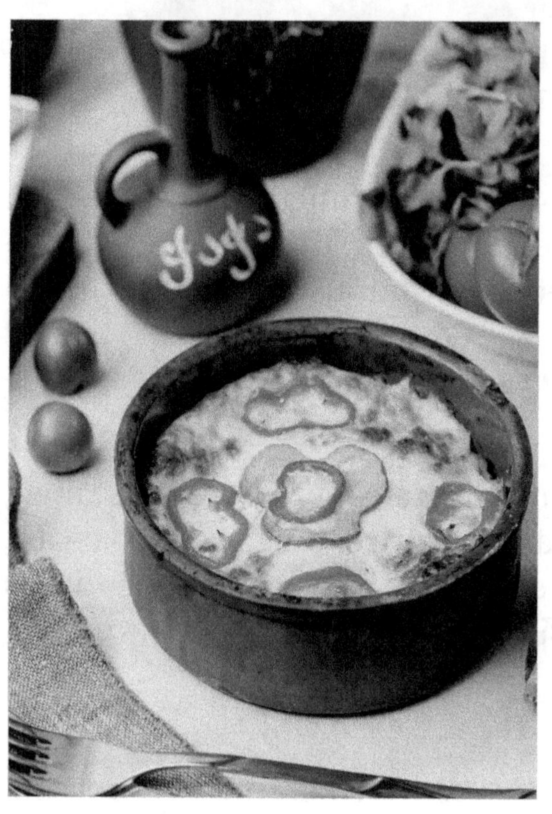

Not all big-batch meals need to be consumed immediately. Consider preparing freezer-friendly dishes that can be stored for longer periods. Soups, stews, and casseroles often freeze well and can be a lifesaver on busy days.

Time and Planning:

Finally, successful big-batch cooking requires careful planning. Dedicate a specific day for meal prep, create a menu, and organize your tasks efficiently. Having a well-organized plan will save time, reduce stress, and ensure that you have a variety of healthy meals readily available throughout the week.

In summary, big-batch cooking for a Healthy Meal Prep Cookbook requires a thoughtful selection of ingredients, proper equipment, and meticulous planning. With the right foundation, you can streamline your cooking process, save time, and enjoy delicious, nutritious meals every day.

Dose the Nutrition Changed?

When it comes to meal prep and cooking, the nutrition of prepared dishes can be influenced by several factors. Let's delve into how the nutrition of prepared dishes might change and what considerations are crucial for maintaining a healthy meal prep routine.

Cooking Methods:

The method of cooking plays a significant role in determining the nutritional content of a dish. Grilling, baking, steaming, and sautéing are generally considered healthier options compared to deep-frying. These methods help preserve the nutrients in the ingredients, ensuring that the prepared meals are rich in essential vitamins and minerals.

Ingredient Choices:

The selection of ingredients is a key factor in the nutritional profile of a meal. In a Healthy Meal Prep Cookbook, the emphasis is often on whole, nutrient-dense foods. Incorporating a variety of colorful vegetables, lean proteins, whole grains, and healthy fats can contribute to a well-balanced and nutritious meal. Choosing organic, locally sourced, or seasonal ingredients can also enhance the overall nutritional quality of the dishes.

Portion Control:

Proper portion control is essential for maintaining a healthy balance of nutrients. Even if the ingredients are nutritious, consuming excessively large portions can lead to an imbalance in calorie intake. A well-designed Healthy Meal Prep Cookbook would likely include guidance on portion sizes to help individuals manage their caloric intake while still enjoying a satisfying and nutritious meal.

Storage and Preservation:

The way meals are stored can impact their nutritional content. For instance, freezing and reheating can cause some loss of water-soluble vitamins such as vitamin C, but the overall impact is often minimal. Using proper storage containers, refrigerating perishable items promptly, and following recommended storage times can help maintain the freshness and nutritional value of prepared meals.

Balanced Macronutrients:

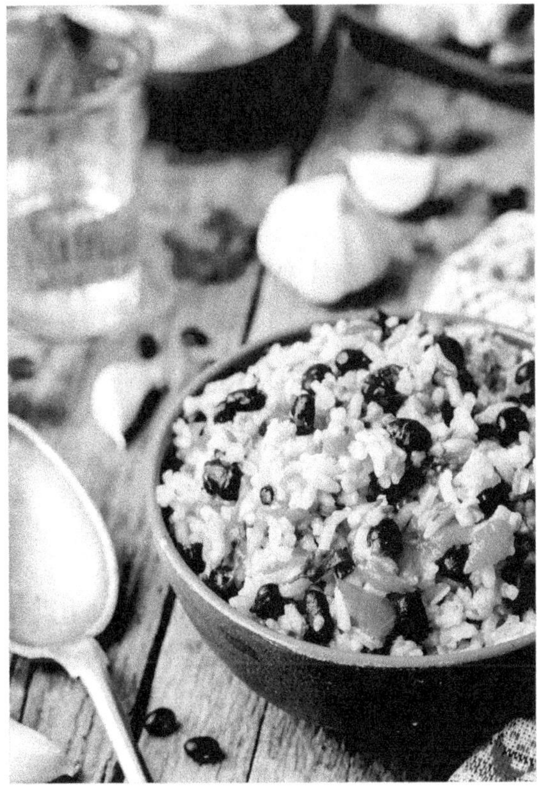

A healthy meal should provide a balanced mix of macronutrients—carbohydrates, proteins, and fats. A well-designed Healthy Meal Prep Cookbook would likely aim to create recipes that offer a balance of these macronutrients to support overall health. For example, incorporating sources of healthy fats like avocados or nuts, lean proteins such as chicken or tofu, and complex carbohydrates like quinoa or sweet potatoes.

Mindful Seasoning:

The way dishes are seasoned can impact both their taste and nutritional content. While minimizing the use of excessive salt

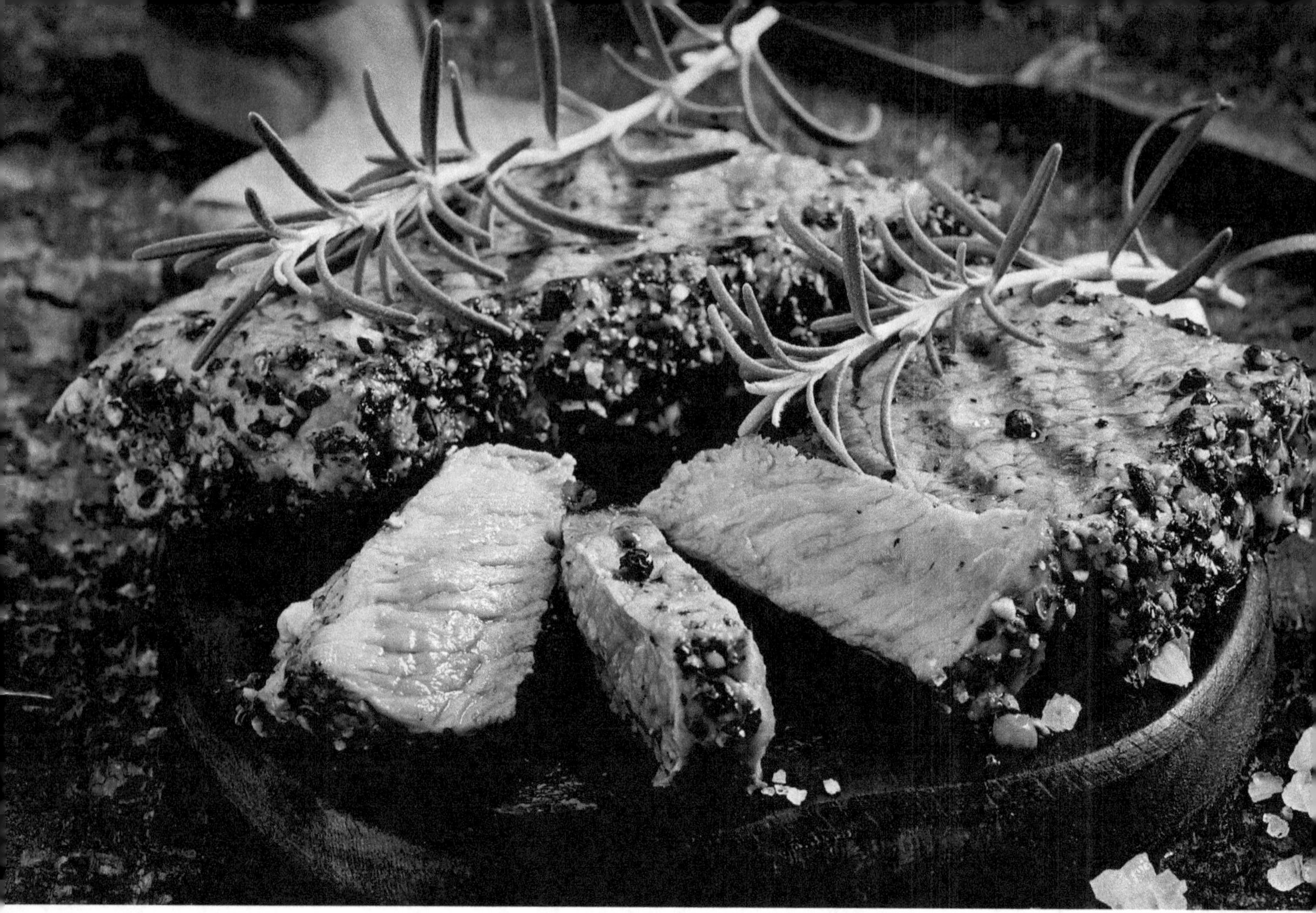

and sugar is a common goal in healthy meal preparation, incorporating herbs, spices, and other flavor-enhancing ingredients can add depth and richness without compromising nutritional value.

Adaptability for Dietary Needs:

A good Healthy Meal Prep Cookbook recognizes that individuals may have different dietary needs or preferences. Whether someone is following a specific diet (e.g., vegetarian, vegan, paleo) or has dietary restrictions (e.g., gluten-free, dairy-free), a well-crafted cookbook provides a variety of options to cater to diverse nutritional requirements.

In conclusion, the nutrition of prepared dishes can be positively influenced by mindful choices in cooking methods, ingredient selection, portion control, storage practices, and an overall commitment to balance and variety. A Healthy Meal Prep Cookbook serves as a valuable guide, empowering individuals to make informed decisions about their nutrition while enjoying delicious and satisfying meals.

How to Freeze and Store?

Freezing and storing meals properly is crucial when it comes to meal prepping, especially for a Healthy Meal Prep Cookbook. This ensures that the nutritional value, taste, and overall quality of the meals are preserved until you're ready to enjoy them. Here's a comprehensive guide on how to freeze and store your healthy meal preps:

Choose Freezer-Friendly Recipes:

Start by selecting recipes that are suitable for freezing. Not all dishes freeze well, and certain ingredients may not maintain their texture after thawing. Opt for recipes that include ingredients like whole grains, lean proteins, and vegetables, as these tend to freeze better.

Allow Meals to Cool:

Before placing your meals in the freezer, make sure they are completely cool. Rapid temperature changes can affect the texture of certain foods. Allow hot dishes to come to room temperature before transferring them to the freezer.

Use Freezer-Safe Containers:

Invest in high-quality, freezer-safe containers. These can be a variety of materials, including glass, plastic, or aluminum. Make sure the containers have a tight-fitting lid to prevent freezer burn and the absorption of odors from the freezer.

Portion Control:

Divide your meals into individual or family-sized portions before freezing. This not only makes it easier to thaw and reheat the right amount but also helps in maintaining the quality of the food. Consider using silicone muffin cups or ice cube trays for smaller portions.

Label and Date:

Proper labeling is essential for keeping track of what's in your freezer and ensuring that you use meals within their optimal timeframe. Include the name of the dish, the date it was prepared, and any reheating instructions. Use a permanent marker or labels that adhere well to frozen surfaces.

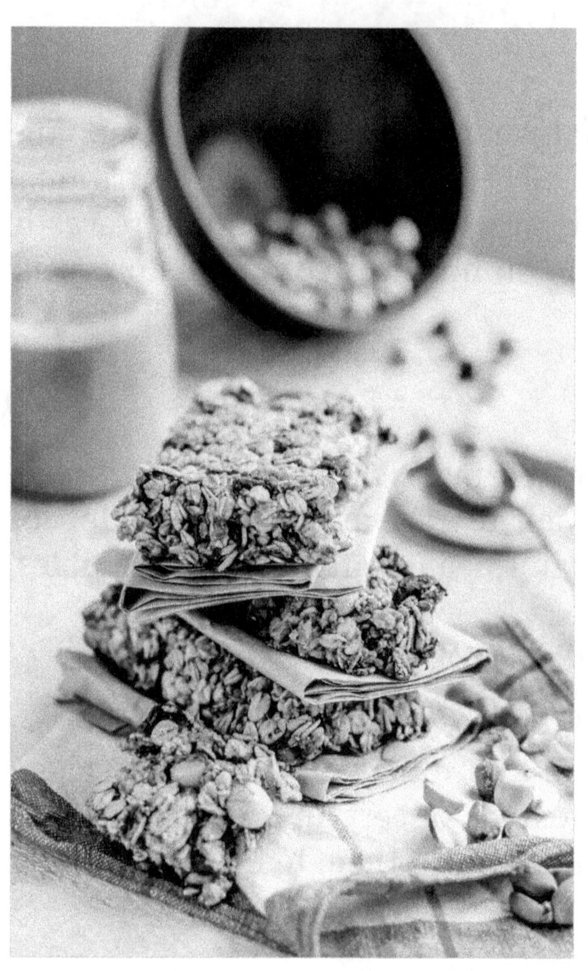

Remove Air from Containers:

The less air inside the container, the better your meals will freeze. Air can lead to freezer burn, which affects the taste and texture of food. Consider using vacuum-sealing bags or containers to remove excess air.

Leave Room for Expansion:

Liquids expand when frozen, so be sure to leave some space at the top of your containers to account for this expansion. For soups and stews, leave about an inch of space to prevent spills and breakage.

Flash Freezing:

For items like fruits, vegetables, or individually portioned proteins, consider flash freezing before placing them in a larger container. This involves spreading items on a baking sheet and freezing them individually before transferring to a larger bag or container. This prevents items from clumping together.

Store Properly in the Freezer:

Organize your freezer to maintain proper airflow and temperature distribution. Place newer items towards the back and rotate older items to the front. This helps ensure that you use the oldest items first.

Keep an Inventory:

Maintain a freezer inventory to keep track of what you have. Regularly update the list as you add or remove items. This helps in preventing food waste and ensures you use up your frozen meals before they lose their quality.

By following these steps, you can freeze and store your healthy meal preps effectively, allowing you to enjoy nutritious and delicious meals with the convenience of prepping ahead of time.

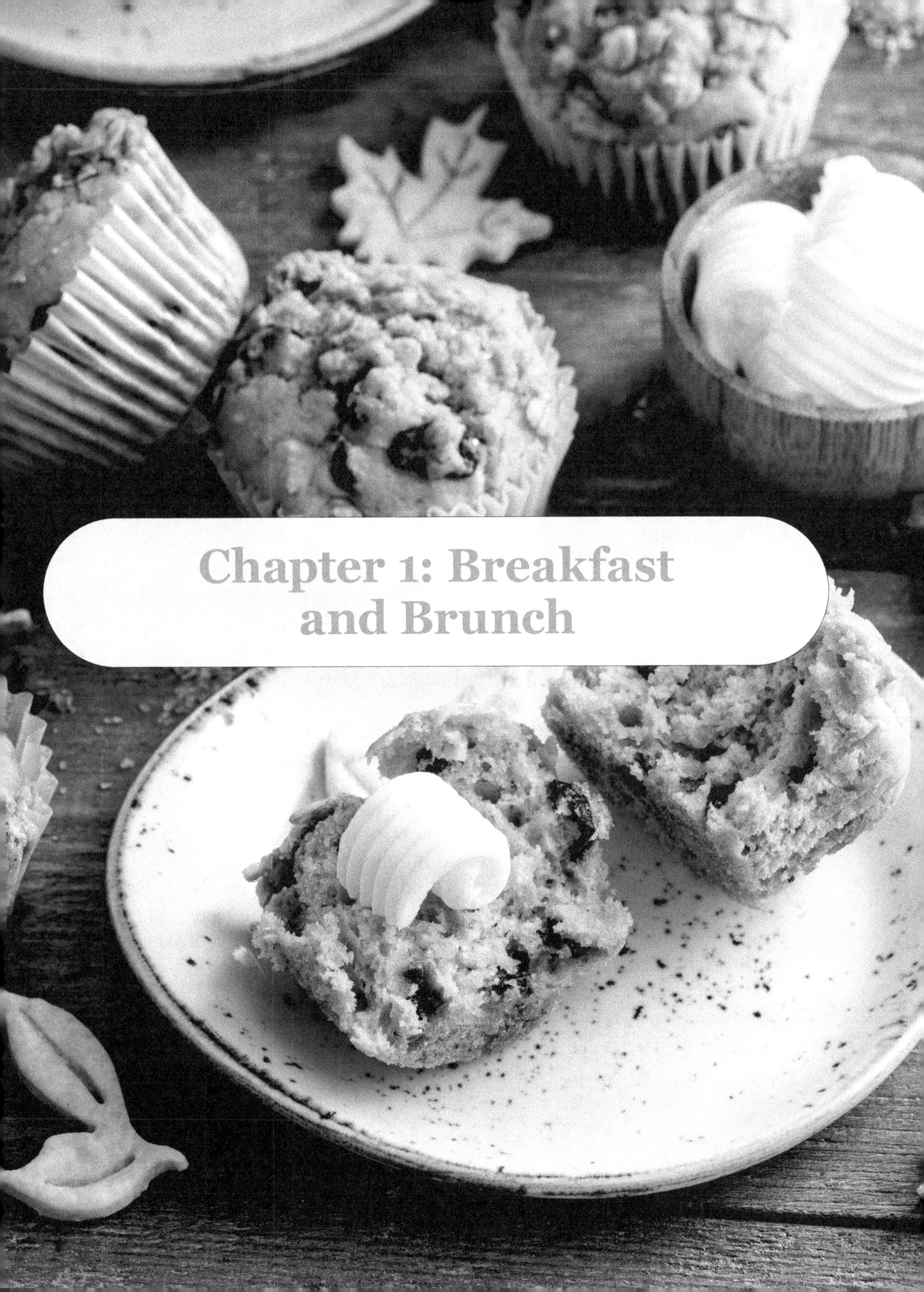
Chapter 1: Breakfast
and Brunch

Oatmeal Breakfast Cookies

Prep Time: 10 Minutes   Cook Time: 20 Minutes   Serves: 12

Ingredients:

- 2 tablespoons ground flaxseed + 5 tablespoons warm water
- 1 cup oat flour, made from 1¼ cups whole rolled oats
- 1 cup additional whole rolled oats
- ½ cup almond flour
- zest of 1 lemon, about ½ tablespoon
- ½ teaspoon baking powder
- ½ teaspoon baking soda
- ½ teaspoon cinnamon
- ½ teaspoon sea salt
- ½ cup creamy natural almond butter
- ¼ cup coconut oil, melted
- ½ cup maple syrup
- ⅓ cup walnuts
- ¾ cup fresh blueberries

Directions:

1. Preheat the oven to 350°F and line a large baking sheet with parchment paper.
2. In a small bowl, combine the flaxseed and warm water and set aside to thicken for 5 minutes.
3. In a large bowl, stir together the oat flour, the additional 1 cup rolled oats, almond flour, lemon zest, baking powder, baking soda, cinnamon, and salt.
4. In a medium bowl, combine the almond butter, coconut oil, and maple syrup and stir well to incorporate. Stir in the flaxseed mixture.
5. Add the wet ingredients to the bowl of dry ingredients and fold in just until combined. Fold in the walnuts and blueberries.
6. Scoop ¼ cup of batter for each cookie onto the baking sheet. Bake 20 to 24 minutes, or until browned around the edges. Cool on the pan for 5 to 10 minutes and then transfer to a wire rack to finish cooling. If you take them off the sheet too soon, the cookies may fall apart.
7. When cookies are completely cool, they can be stored in an airtight container or frozen.

Nutritional Value (Amount per Serving):

Calories: 221; Fat: 13.19; Carb: 25.76; Protein: 5.27

Overnight Oats

Prep Time: 10 Minutes   Cook Time: 10 Minutes   Serves:1

Ingredients:

- ½ cup whole rolled oats
- 1 tablespoon chia seeds
- ½ teaspoon maple syrup, plus more for serving
- Pinch of sea salt
- ¼ cup whole milk Greek yogurt, optional
- ⅔ cup unsweetened almond milk

Directions:

1. Make the base recipe: In a Mason jar or other lidded jar, place the oats, chia seeds, maple syrup, salt, and Greek yogurt, if using. Add the almond milk and stir until the mixture is well combined and there are no clumps of chia seeds at the bottom of the jar. Cover and refrigerate overnight, or for up to 5 days.
2. In the morning, top with your desired toppings and serve with drizzles of maple syrup.

Nutritional Value (Amount per Serving):

Calories: 291; Fat: 10.38; Carb: 55.49; Protein: 12.93

Tropical Overnight Oats

Prep Time: 10 Minutes   Cook Time: 7 Hours 50 Minutes   Serves: 1

Ingredients:

- ½ cup rolled oats (see Tip)
- ¾ cup unsweetened coconut milk beverage
- ¼ cup diced pineapple
- 1 tablespoon chopped unsweetened dried mango
- 1 ½ teaspoons chia seeds
- 1 ½ teaspoons unsweetened shredded coconut

Directions:

1. Combine oats, coconut milk, pineapple, mango and chia seeds in a small bowl or jar. Cover and refrigerate overnight.
2. Top with coconut before serving.
3. Refrigerate for up to 5 days.

Nutritional Value (Amount per Serving):

Calories: 649; Fat: 50.9; Carb: 59.53; Protein: 15.07

Veggie Frittata Muffins

Prep Time: 10 Minutes   Cook Time: 20 Minutes   Serves: 12

Ingredients:

- 8 large eggs
- ⅓ cup unsweetened almond milk
- 1 garlic clove, minced
- ¼ teaspoon Dijon mustard
- ½ teaspoon sea salt
- freshly ground black pepper
- 2 to 4 tablespoons chopped fresh dill
- 2 small kale leaves, finely shredded
- 1 cup halved cherry tomatoes
- ¼ cup scallions
- ⅓ cup crumbled feta

Directions:

1. Preheat the oven to 350°F and brush a nonstick muffin pan with olive oil or nonstick cooking spray.
2. In a large bowl, whisk together the eggs, milk, garlic, dijon mustard, most of the dill (reserve a little for garnish), salt and pepper. Pour just a bit of the egg mixture into the bottom of each muffin cup. Divide the kale, tomatoes, scallions and feta into each cup, then pour the remaining egg mixture on top.
3. Bake for 20 to 22 minutes or until the eggs are set. Season with salt and pepper to taste, and garnish with the remaining dill. Store any remaining frittatas in the fridge for up to 2 days.

Nutritional Value (Amount per Serving):

Calories: 58; Fat: 4.29; Carb: 2.26; Protein: 2.89

Homemade Granola

Prep Time: 10 Minutes   Cook Time: 30 Minutes   Serves: 4-6

Ingredients:

- 2 cups whole rolled oats
- 1/2 cup chopped walnuts, (or almonds, or a mix of both)
- 1/2 cup coconut flakes, optional
- 2 teaspoons cinnamon
- 1/2 teaspoon sea salt
- 2 tablespoons melted coconut oil

- 1/4 cup maple syrup
- 2 tablespoons creamy almond butter
- 1/3 cup dried cranberries, optional

Directions:

1. Preheat the oven to 300°F and line a baking sheet with parchment paper.
2. In a medium bowl, combine the oats, walnuts, coconut flakes, if using, cinnamon, and salt. Drizzle in the coconut oil and maple syrup and add the almond butter. Stir until combined. Scoop the granola onto the baking sheet and press the mixture into a 1-inch-thick oval. This will encourage clumping.
3. Bake for 15 minutes, rotate the pan halfway, and use a fork to gently break the granola apart just a bit. Bake for 15 minutes, or until golden brown. Sprinkle with dried cranberries, if desired. Let cool for 15 minutes before serving or storing.

Nutritional Value (Amount per Serving):

Calories: 322; Fat: 19.27; Carb: 45.27; Protein: 9.38

Pumpkin Muffins

Prep Time: 15 Minutes   Cook Time: 20 Minutes   Serves: 12

Ingredients:

- 1 cup pumpkin puree
- 2 large eggs
- ⅔ cup unsweetened almond milk
- ⅓ cup melted coconut oil, or vegetable oil
- ⅓ cup maple syrup
- 1 tablespoon apple cider vinegar
- 1 teaspoon vanilla extract
- 1 cup all-purpose flour
- ¾ cup whole wheat flour
- 1 tablespoon pumpkin pie spice
- 1 teaspoon baking powder
- ½ teaspoon baking soda
- ½ teaspoon sea salt

Directions:

1. Preheat the oven to 350°F and lightly grease or spray a 12-cup muffin tin.
2. In a large bowl, combine the pumpkin puree, eggs, almond milk, oil, maple syrup, vinegar, and vanilla and whisk until combined.
3. In a medium bowl, whisk together the flours, pumpkin pie spice, baking powder, baking soda, and salt.

4. Add the dry ingredients to the wet ingredients and stir until just combined.
5. Use a ⅓-cup measuring scoop to divide the batter into the muffin tin. Bake for 18 to 20 minutes or until a toothpick inserted comes out clean.
6. Let the muffins cool in the pan for 10 minutes before transferring them to a wire rack to cool completely.

Nutritional Value (Amount per Serving):

Calories: 213; Fat: 12.09; Carb: 22.67; Protein: 5.57

Healthy Banana Bread

Prep Time: 10 Minutes   Cook Time: 45 Minutes   Serves: 8

Ingredients:

- 2 very ripe bananas, mashed (1 cup)
- ½ cup coconut sugar, or regular sugar
- ¾ cup almond milk, or any milk
- ⅓ cup extra-virgin olive oil, more for brushing
- 1 teaspoon vanilla extract
- 1 teaspoon apple cider vinegar
- 1½ cups whole wheat pastry flour
- ½ cup almond flour
- 2 teaspoons baking powder
- ¼ teaspoon baking soda
- ½ teaspoon sea salt
- ½ teaspoon cinnamon
- ¼ teaspoon nutmeg
- ½ cup chopped walnuts
- 2 tablespoons chopped walnuts
- 1 1/2 tablespoon rolled oats

Directions:

1. Preheat the oven to 350°F and brush a 9x5-inch loaf pan with a bit of olive oil.
2. In a large bowl, combine the mashed bananas with the sugar, almond milk, olive oil, vanilla, and apple cider vinegar and whisk until combined.
3. In a medium bowl combine the flours, baking powder, baking soda, salt, cinnamon, and nutmeg.
4. Add the dry ingredients to the bowl with the wet ingredients, and stir until just combined, then fold in the walnuts. Pour into the prepared pan and sprinkle with the chopped walnuts and oats.
5. Bake for 42 to 50 minutes, or until a toothpick inserted in the middle comes out clean.

Calories: 181; Fat: 8.92; Carb: 24.56; Protein: 3.35

Overnight Oats Blueberry Smoothie Bowl

Prep Time: 10 Minutes   Cook Time: 8 Hours   Serves: 2

Ingredients:

- 1 cup rolled oats
- 1 ¼ cups unsweetened vanilla-flavored almond milk, divided
- 1 frozen banana, chopped
- 1 cup blueberries
- 1 teaspoon vanilla extract
- 1 teaspoon maple syrup, or to taste
- 2 tablespoons flaked coconut
- 1 tablespoon fresh blueberries
- 1 teaspoon chia seeds

Directions:

1. Combine oats and 2/3 cup almond milk in a bowl; cover and refrigerate until milk is absorbed by oats, 8 hours to overnight.
2. Combine oats-almond milk mixture, remaining almond milk, banana, blueberries, vanilla, and maple syrup in a blender; blend until smooth.
3. Pour smoothie into 2 bowls, then top with coconut, blueberries, and chia seeds.

Nutritional Value (Amount per Serving):

Calories: 507; Fat: 7.79; Carb: 120.29; Protein: 12.53

Avocado and Feta Egg White Omelet

Prep Time: 5 Minutes   Cook Time: 5 Minutes   Serves: 1

Ingredients:

- ½ cup egg whites
- 1 teaspoon paprika
- ½ tablespoon olive oil
- 3 leaves fresh basil
- ½ avocado, sliced
- 2 tablespoons crumbled feta cheese

Directions:

1. Mix egg whites and paprika together in a bowl.
2. Heat olive oil in a small skillet over medium heat. Pour in egg white mixture; cook for 1 minute. Place basil leaves over egg whites. Cook until egg white starts to firm up, about 1 minute. Spread avocado on top and

sprinkle with feta cheese. Cook for 3 minutes. Fold in half to form the omelet.

Calories: 1083; Fat: 85.89; Carb: 23.01; Protein: 58.26

Baby Spinach Omelet

Prep Time: 5 Minutes   Cook Time:10 Minutes   Serves: 1

Ingredients:

- 2 eggs
- 1 cup torn baby spinach leaves
- 1 ½ tablespoons grated Parmesan cheese
- ¼ teaspoon onion powder
- ⅛ teaspoon ground nutmeg
- salt and pepper to taste

Directions:

1. Beat eggs in a bowl, and stir in baby spinach and Parmesan cheese. Season with onion powder, nutmeg, salt, and pepper.
2. Spray a small skillet with cooking spray and place over medium heat. Once warm, add in the egg mixture and cook until partially set, about 3 minutes. Flip with a spatula, and continue cooking, 2 to 3 minutes.
3. Reduce heat to low and continue cooking, 2 to 3 minutes, or until omelet reaches desired doneness.

Nutritional Value (Amount per Serving):

Calories: 319; Fat: 21.69; Carb: 9.04; Protein: 21.9

Perfect Breakfast

Prep Time: 10 Minutes   Cook Time: 5 Minutes   Serves: 1

Ingredients:

- 2 teaspoons butter
- 2 eggs
- 1 slice sourdough bread, toasted
- Dijon mustard
- ½ avocado - peeled, pitted, and sliced
- 2 tablespoons grated Parmesan cheese, or more to taste

Directions:

1. Melt butter in a skillet over medium heat. Add eggs and cook until whites are mostly firm. Break yolks and continue cooking until eggs are set and no longer runny, 2 to 3 more minutes.
2. Spread one side of toasted sourdough with Dijon mustard. Arrange avocado

slices on bread and top with cooked eggs. Sprinkle with Parmesan cheese.

Nutritional Value (Amount per Serving):

Calories: 589; Fat: 45.5; Carb: 22.47; Protein: 25.01

Soft Hard-Boiled Eggs

Prep Time: 3 Minutes   Cook Time: 9 Minutes   Serves: 6

Ingredients:

- 1 ¼ cups water
- 6 large cold eggs

Directions:

1. Place water into a 3-quart saucepan with a lid. Place over high heat and bring to a low boil. Carefully place eggs in the water. Cover pan immediately, reduce heat to medium-high, and cook for 9 1/2 minutes.
2. Remove pan from heat and cool eggs down with cold running water, tipping out the water, and continuing to run cold water over the eggs until they are cool.

Nutritional Value (Amount per Serving):

Calories: 55; Fat: 4.51; Carb: 0.61; Protein: 2.7

Coconut Overnight Oats

Prep Time: 5 Minutes   Cook Time: 8 Hours   Serves:1

Ingredients:

- ⅓ cup old-fashioned oats
- ⅓ cup coconut milk beverage
- ¼ cup nonfat vanilla Greek yogurt
- ½ tablespoon chia seeds
- 1 ½ tablespoons unsweetened shredded coconut, divided
- ½ tablespoon cacao nibs
- ½ tablespoon sliced almonds

Directions:

1. Combine oats, coconut milk beverage, Greek yogurt, chia seeds, and 1 tablespoon coconut flakes in an 8-ounce Mason jar. Stir until well combined, and cover with a lid. Refrigerate for 8 hours, or overnight.
2. Top with ½ tablespoon coconut flakes, cacao nibs, and almonds flakes when ready to serve. Stir and enjoy.

Nutritional Value (Amount per Serving):

Calories: 486; Fat: 34.78; Carb: 43.25; Protein: 16.18

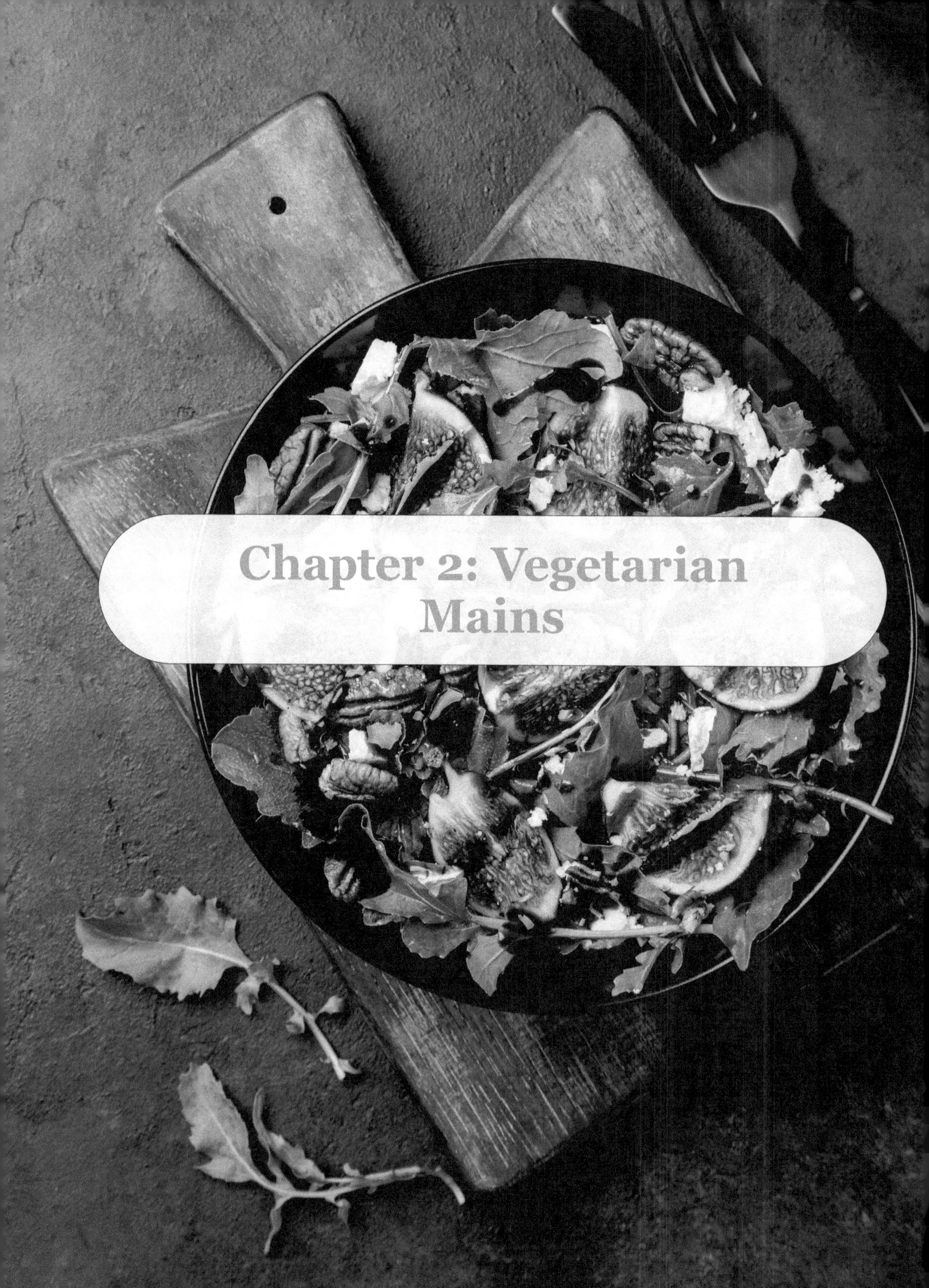
Chapter 2: Vegetarian Mains

Vegan Quinoa and Guac Bowl

Prep Time: 15 Minutes   Cook Time: 30 Minutes   Serves: 3

Ingredients:

- 3 tablespoons olive oil, divided
- 1 (14 ounce) package extra-firm tofu, drained
- ½ teaspoon salt
- black pepper to taste
- 1 ½ teaspoons onion powder
- 1 ½ teaspoons garlic powder
- ½ teaspoon ground turmeric
- 1 tablespoon fresh lemon juice
- 1 tablespoon olive oil
- 1 cup finely diced red onion
- 2 jalapeno peppers, seeded and chopped
- ½ teaspoon salt
- 3 cloves garlic, minced
- 2 cups chopped tomatoes
- 1 ½ teaspoons cumin
- ¼ cup chopped fresh cilantro
- 1 tablespoon fresh lemon juice
- 1 (15.5 ounce) can no-salt-added black beans, drained and rinsed
- 1 ½ cups cooked hash brown potatoes
- 1 avocado - peeled, pitted and sliced
- 1 teaspoon fresh lemon juice
- ¼ cup chopped fresh cilantro
- 1 teaspoon hot sauce, or to taste

Directions:

1. Preheat a large, heavy skillet over medium-high heat. Add 2 tablespoons oil. Break tofu apart over skillet into bite-size pieces, sprinkle with salt and pepper, then cook, stirring frequently with a thin metal spatula, until liquid cooks out and tofu browns, about 10 minutes. (If you notice liquid collecting in pan, increase heat to evaporate water.) Be sure to get under the tofu when you stir, scraping the bottom of the pan where the good, crispy stuff is and keeping it from sticking.

2. Add onion and garlic powders, turmeric, juice, and remaining tablespoon oil and toss to coat. Cook 5 minutes.

3. Preheat a heavy-bottomed saucepan over medium-high heat. Add oil. Cook onion and jalapenos with a pinch of salt, stirring, until translucent, about 5 minutes. Add garlic and cook, stirring, until fragrant, about 30 seconds. Add tomatoes, cumin, and remaining salt, and cook, stirring, until

tomatoes become saucy, about 5 minutes. Add cilantro and lemon juice. Let cilantro wilt in. Add beans and heat through, stirring occasionally, about 2 minutes. Taste for salt and seasoning.

4. Spoon some hash browns into each bowl, followed by a scoop of beans and a scoop of scramble.
5. When ready to eat, top with avocado, a squeeze of fresh lemon juice, and a sprinkle of cilantro. Serve with hot sauce.
6. Refrigerate in covered containers for up to 4 days.

Nutritional Value (Amount per Serving):

Calories: 574; Fat: 36.29; Carb: 49.94; Protein: 20.13

Broccoli Cauliflower Chickpea Bowl

Prep Time: 15 Minutes   Cook Time: 30 Minutes   Serves: 5

Ingredients:

- ½ cup cashews
- 4 cups broccoli florets
- 4 cups cauliflower florets
- ½ teaspoon garlic powder
- salt and ground black pepper to taste
- 1 (15 ounce) can chickpeas (garbanzo beans), drained and rinsed
- 2 tablespoons lemon juice
- 1 tablespoon tahini
- ½ teaspoon salt

Directions:

1. Place cashews in a bowl and top with water; soak until softened, 3 to 4 hours.
2. Preheat oven to 400 degrees F. Line 2 baking sheets with parchment paper or spray with cooking spray.
3. Spread broccoli and cauliflower onto 1 baking sheet, and season with garlic powder, salt, and pepper. Spread chickpeas onto the other baking sheet, and season with salt and pepper.
4. Roast in the preheated oven until broccoli, cauliflower, and chickpeas are softened and cooked through, about 30 minutes.
5. Drain cashews. Combine cashews, lemon juice, tahini, and 1/2 teaspoon salt in a blender or food processor; blend until dressing is smooth.
6. Transfer broccoli, cauliflower, and chickpeas to serving bowl. Drizzle dressing over vegetables and chickpeas.
7. Refrigerate in covered containers for up to 4 days.

Nutritional Value (Amount per Serving):

Calories: 278; Fat: 16.87; Carb: 26.68; Protein: 10.1

Vegan Bistro Lunch Box

Prep Time: 5 Minutes   Cook Time: 5 Minutes   Serves: 1

Ingredients:

- ¼ cup hummus
- ½ whole-wheat pita bread, cut into 4 wedges
- 2 tablespoons mixed olives
- 1 Persian cucumber or 1/2 English cucumber, cut into spears
- ¼ large red bell pepper, sliced
- ¼ teaspoon chopped fresh dill

Directions:

1. Arrange hummus, pita, olives, cucumber and bell peppers in a 4-cup divided sealable container. (If desired, the hummus and olives can be kept separate by placing them in silicone baking cups before arranging.) Sprinkle cucumber with dill. Keep refrigerated until ready to use.
2. Refrigerate for up to 1 day.

Nutritional Value (Amount per Serving):

Calories: 196; Fat: 7.86; Carb: 26.81; Protein: 5.99

Slow-Cooker Creamy Lentil Soup Freezer Pack

Prep Time: 25 Minutes   Cook Time: 4 Hours   Serves: 4

Ingredients:

- 1 cup green or brown lentils, picked over and rinsed
- 1 cup chopped onions
- 1 cup diced carrots
- 2 tablespoons finely chopped garlic
- 2 teaspoons ground coriander
- 2 bay leaves
- 1 teaspoon ground cumin
- 1 teaspoon dried oregano
- 1 teaspoon ground pepper
- ¼ teaspoon cayenne pepper
- 4 cups vegetable broth
- 2 cups coarsely chopped spinach
- 1 (15 ounce) can diced tomatoes
- ⅔ cup light coconut milk
- ¼ cup chopped fresh parsley
- 1 tablespoon white-wine vinegar

- ½ teaspoon salt

Directions:

1. To prepare freezer pack: Combine lentils, onions, carrots, garlic, coriander, bay leaves, cumin, oregano, pepper and cayenne in a sealable plastic bag. Seal and freeze for up to 6 months.
2. To prepare soup: Empty the freezer bag into a 6-quart slow-cooker. Add broth. Cover and cook on High for 4 hours or on Low for 8 hours.
3. Discard bay leaves. Transfer half of the soup to a blender and puree. (Use caution when blending hot liquids.) Return the pureed soup to the slow cooker and stir in spinach, tomatoes, coconut milk, parsley, vinegar and salt; heat through.
4. Refrigerate soup for up to 4 days, or freeze for up to 4 months. Reheat before serving.

Nutritional Value (Amount per Serving):

Calories: 195; Fat: 10.6; Carb: 23.2; Protein: 7.19

Vegan Burrito Bowls with Cauliflower Rice

Prep Time: 25 Minutes   Cook Time: 25 Minutes   Serves: 4

Ingredients:

- 1 recipe Tofu Crumbles (see associated recipe)
- 1 (12 ounce) package frozen riced cauliflower
- 4 teaspoons olive oil
- 1 teaspoon no-salt-added taco seasoning
- 1 cup thinly sliced red cabbage
- 1 cup diced avocado
- ½ cup pico de gallo or salsa
- ¼ cup chopped fresh cilantro

Directions:

1. Prepare Tofu Crumbles as directed.
2. While the Tofu Crumbles cook, prepare riced cauliflower according to package directions. Toss with oil and taco seasoning.
3. Divide the cauliflower among 4 single-serving containers with lids. Top each with 1/2 cup Beefless Ground Beef, 1/4 cup each cabbage and avocado, 2 tablespoons pico de gallo (or salsa) and 1 tablespoon cilantro. Seal the containers and refrigerate until ready to eat. Refrigerate for up to 4 days.

Nutritional Value (Amount per Serving):

Calories: 170; Fat: 14.27; Carb: 8.04; Protein: 5.04

Veggistrone

Prep Time: 1 Hour   Cook Time: 45 Minutes   Serves: 10

Ingredients:

- 2 tablespoons extra-virgin olive oil
- 2 cups chopped onions (2 medium)
- 2 cups chopped celery (4 medium stalks)
- 1 cup chopped green bell pepper (1 medium)
- 4 cloves garlic, minced
- 3 cups chopped cabbage
- 3 cups chopped cauliflower (about 1/2 medium)
- 2 cups chopped carrots (4 medium)
- 2 cups green beans, cut into 1-inch pieces, or frozen, thawed
- 8 cups low-sodium vegetable broth or chicken broth
- 2 cups water
- 1 (15 ounce) can tomato sauce
- 1 (14 ounce) can diced tomatoes
- 1 (15 ounce) can kidney or pinto beans, rinsed
- 1 bay leaf
- 4 cups chopped fresh spinach or 1 (10 ounce) package frozen chopped spinach, thawed
- ½ cup thinly sliced fresh basil
- 10 tablespoons freshly grated Parmesan cheese

Directions:

1. Heat oil in a large soup pot or Dutch oven (8-quart or larger) over medium heat. Add onions, celery, bell pepper and garlic; cook, stirring frequently, until softened, 13 to 15 minutes. Add cabbage, cauliflower, carrots and green beans; cook, stirring occasionally, until slightly softened, about 10 minutes.
2. Add broth, water, tomato sauce, tomatoes, beans and bay leaf; cover and bring to a boil. Reduce heat and simmer, partially covered, until the vegetables are tender, 20 to 25 minutes. Stir in spinach and simmer for 10 minutes .
3. Discard the bay leaf. Stir in basil. Top each portion with 1 tablespoon cheese.
4. Prepare through Step 2 and refrigerate for up to 5 days or freeze for up to 6 months; finish Step 3 just before serving.

Nutritional Value (Amount per Serving):

Calories: 250; Fat: 4.16; Carb: 42.14; Protein: 13.86

Prep Time: 35 Minutes   Cook Time: 30 Minutes   Serves: 6

Ingredients:

- 2 tablespoons extra-virgin olive oil
- 8 ounces fresh mixed wild mushrooms (such as oyster and shiitake), sliced
- 1 cup thinly sliced yellow onion
- 1 tablespoon minced garlic
- 2 teaspoons minced fresh thyme
- 1 (5 ounce) package fresh spinach, coarsely chopped
- 8 large eggs
- ⅔ cup whole milk
- 2 teaspoons Dijon mustard
- ½ teaspoon salt
- ½ teaspoon ground pepper
- ¾ cup shredded Gruyère cheese

Directions:

1. Preheat oven to 325 degrees F. Heat oil in a large nonstick skillet over medium-high heat. Add mushrooms in an even layer; cook, undisturbed, until browned on the bottom, about 4 minutes. Stir and continue to cook, stirring occasionally, until browned all over, about 5 minutes. Add onion; cook, stirring occasionally, until beginning to soften, about 4 minutes. Stir in garlic and thyme; cook, stirring, until fragrant, about 2 minutes. Add spinach; cook, stirring constantly, until just wilted, about 2 minutes. Remove from heat.
2. Whisk eggs, milk, Dijon, salt and pepper in a large bowl. Stir in cheese and the mushroom mixture. Coat a standard 12-cup muffin tin with cooking spray. Divide the mixture among the prepared muffin cups. Bake, uncovered, until puffed and set, about 30 minutes. Remove from the pan and refrigerate for up to 3 days.

Nutritional Value (Amount per Serving):

Calories: 232; Fat: 15.14; Carb: 14.61; Protein: 10.79

Prep Time: 15 Minutes   Cook Time: 40 Minutes   Serves: 4

Ingredients:

- 1 (15 ounce) can pinto beans, rinsed and drained
- 2 ½ cups water

- 2 cups quinoa
- ½ teaspoon kosher salt
- 1 tablespoon olive oil
- 1 red bell pepper, sliced
- 1 yellow bell pepper, sliced
- ½ teaspoon ground black pepper
- 4 cups lettuce leaves
- 1 cup vegan shredded cheese blend
- 1 avocado - peeled, pitted, and sliced
- ¼ cup vegan sour cream

Directions:

1. Heat pinto beans in a saucepan over low heat until hot, 5 to 7 minutes.
2. Bring water, quinoa, and salt to a boil in a saucepan and simmer until quinoa is tender and water is absorbed, 15 to 20 minutes. Remove from heat and set aside to cool, about 10 minutes.
3. Heat olive oil in a skillet over medium heat. Add red bell pepper, yellow bell pepper, and black pepper; cook and stir until bell peppers are softened but still crisp, about 10 minutes.
4. Toss quinoa, pinto beans, and lettuce together in a bowl. Top with pepper mixture, vegan cheese, avocado, and vegan sour cream.

Nutritional Value (Amount per Serving):

Calories: 650; Fat: 26.69; Carb: 79.12; Protein: 26.66

Roasted Veggie Buddha Bowl

Prep Time: 25 Minutes   Cook Time: 42 Minutes   Serves: 2

Ingredients:

- 1 cup water
- ½ cup bulgur
- 1 sweet potato, peeled and cut into 1-inch cubes
- 4 teaspoons olive oil, divided
- salt and ground black pepper to taste
- ½ pound fennel bulb, trimmed and cut into 1-inch cubes
- 1 small red onion, cut into 1-inch pieces
- 1 red bell pepper, cut into 1-inch strips
- 1 (8 ounce) package tempeh, cut into 1-inch pieces
- ½ teaspoon curry powder
- 2 teaspoons coconut oil
- ¼ cup fresh squeezed orange juice
- 2 tablespoons olive oil

- 2 teaspoons red wine vinegar
- ½ teaspoon curry powder
- ¼ teaspoon salt
- ¼ teaspoon ground black pepper
- 2 tablespoons raw pumpkin seeds (pepitas)

1. Preheat oven to 400 degrees F. Line a baking sheet with parchment paper.
2. Bring water and bulgur to a boil in a saucepan; cover and reduce heat to medium-low. Simmer until water is absorbed and bulgur is soft, about 12 minutes. Keep warm.
3. Place sweet potato in a bowl and drizzle 1 teaspoon olive oil over it; season with salt and pepper. Toss to coat. Transfer sweet potato to the prepared baking sheet, placing in 1 row. Place fennel in the same bowl, add 1 teaspoon olive oil, and season with salt and pepper. Toss to coat and place fennel next to sweet potato, keeping each separate.
4. Roast in the preheated oven for 10 minutes. Place red onion in the same bowl; add 1 teaspoon olive oil, and season with salt and pepper. Toss to coat and place on the baking sheet with sweet potato and fennel, keeping them separate. Place red bell pepper in the same bowl; add 1 teaspoon olive oil, and season with salt and pepper. Toss to coat and place on the baking sheet next to the onion.
5. Roast in the oven until all the vegetables are cooked to desired doneness, 10 to 15 minutes.
6. Place tempeh in a bowl and season with 1/2 teaspoon curry powder, tossing to coat.
7. Heat coconut oil in a skillet over medium-high heat; saute tempeh, turning occasionally, until all sides are evenly browned, about 10 minutes.
8. Whisk orange juice, 2 tablespoons olive oil, red wine vinegar, 1/2 teaspoon curry powder, 1/4 teaspoon salt, and 1/4 teaspoon pepper in a small bowl until dressing is smooth.
9. Divide bulgur between 2 bowls. Place half of sweet potato, fennel, red onion, and red bell pepper around bulgur; top each with 1 tablespoon pumpkin seeds. Drizzle dressing over each bowl.

Nutritional Value (Amount per Serving):

Calories: 651; Fat: 43.83; Carb: 45.99; Protein: 29.29

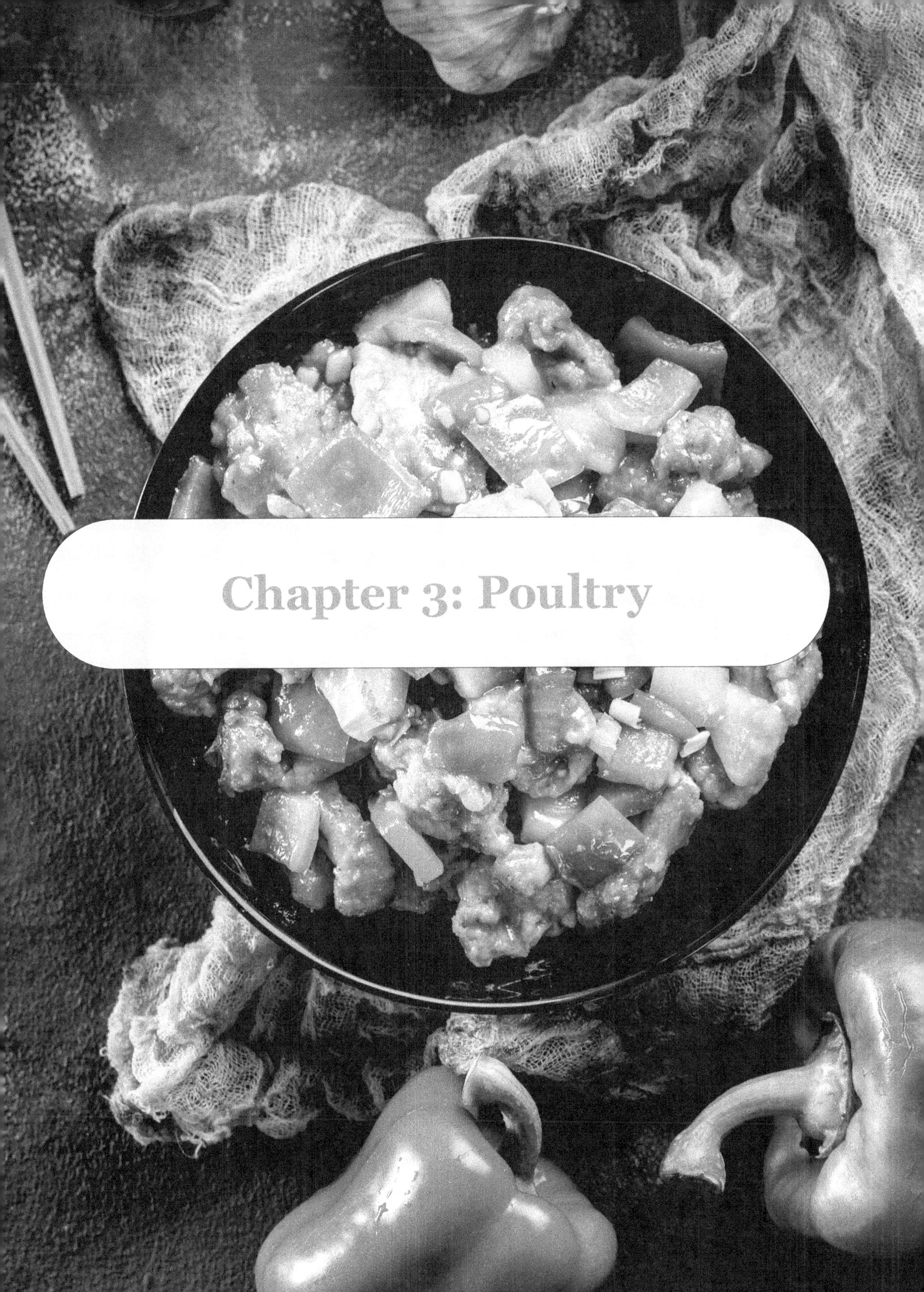

Chapter 3: Poultry

Meal-Prep Chili-Lime Chicken Bowls

Prep Time: 25 Minutes   Cook Time: 5 Minutes   Serves: 4

Ingredients:

- 1 cup cooked quinoa
- 1 cup cooked brown rice
- 1 pound cooked Chili-Lime Chicken (see Associated recipe)
- 1 cup julienned jicama
- 1 cup frozen corn, thawed
- 1 cup pico de gallo
- 1 avocado, diced
- ½ cup chopped fresh cilantro
- Lime wedges
- Hot sauce, such as Cholula

Directions:

1. Combine quinoa and rice; divide among 4 single-serving containers with lids. Top with chicken, jicama, corn, pico de gallo and cilantro, dividing evenly. Seal the containers and refrigerate for up to 4 days.
2. Serve with diced avocado, lime wedges and hot sauce.

Nutritional Value (Amount per Serving):

Calories: 879; Fat: 55.99; Carb: 63.99; Protein: 30.87

Meal-Prep Curried Chicken & Chili-Lime Chicken

Prep Time: 5 Minutes   Cook Time:5 Minutes   Serves: 4

Ingredients:

- 1 cup cooked brown rice
- 1 cup cooked quinoa
- 1 pound cooked Curried Chicken
- ¼ cup chopped fresh cilantro
- ¼ cup thinly sliced scallions

Directions:

1. Combine rice and quinoa; divide among 4 single-serving containers with lids. Top with chicken, cilantro and scallions, dividing evenly.
2. Seal the containers and refrigerate for up to 4 days.

Nutritional Value (Amount per Serving):

Calories: 735; Fat: 49.76; Carb: 40.45; Protein: 29.25

Cheesy Chicken Meatballs

Prep Time: 20 Minutes   Cook Time: 20 Minutes   Serves: 5

Ingredients:

- 1 pound ground chicken
- 2 eggs, lightly beaten
- ¼ cup roasted garlic light cream cheese
- ¼ cup grated Parmesan cheese
- 1 tablespoon dry bread crumbs
- 1 teaspoon crushed red pepper flakes
- 1 tablespoon Italian seasoning
- 1 tablespoon garlic powder
- 1 ½ tablespoons vegetable oil
- 1 teaspoon salt
- 1 teaspoon ground black pepper

Directions:

1. Preheat an oven to 450 degrees F. Line a rimmed baking sheet with aluminum foil, and spray with cooking spray.
2. Combine the chicken, eggs, cream cheese, Parmesan cheese, bread crumbs, red pepper flakes, Italian seasoning, garlic powder, vegetable oil, salt, and pepper in a large bowl; mix well. Form mixture into 20 meatballs; place on prepared pan.
3. Bake in center of preheated oven until juices run clear, 17 to 18 minutes. An instant-read thermometer inserted into the center should read at least 165 degrees F. Seal the containers and refrigerate for up to 3 days.

Nutritional Value (Amount per Serving):

Calories: 298; Fat: 20.23; Carb: 6.65; Protein: 22.62

Moroccan-Inspired Chicken & Sweet Potato Soup

Prep Time: 40 Minutes   Cook Time: 30 Minutes   Serves: 8

Ingredients:

- 2 tablespoons extra-virgin olive oil
- 1 cup chopped onion
- 2 large cloves garlic, minced
- 1 ½ teaspoons ground cumin
- ½ teaspoon ground cinnamon
- ¼ teaspoon cayenne pepper
- 8 cups low-sodium chicken broth

- 2 pounds bone-in chicken breasts, skin removed
- 3 cups diced sweet potato
- 2 cups diced red bell pepper
- 2 cups green beans (1-inch pieces), fresh or frozen (thawed)
- 1 (15 ounce) can chickpeas, rinsed
- 1 ¼ teaspoons salt
- ½ teaspoon ground pepper
- 1 teaspoon harissa, or to taste

Directions:

1. Heat oil in a large pot over medium heat. Add onion and garlic and cook, stirring occasionally, until softened, 2 to 3 minutes. Add cumin, cinnamon and cayenne; cook, stirring, for 1 minute. Add broth and chicken. Cover, increase heat to high and bring to a simmer. Uncover and cook, turning the chicken occasionally, until an instant-read thermometer inserted into the thickest part without touching bone registers 165 degrees F, 20 to 22 minutes. Skim any foam from the surface as the chicken cooks. Transfer the chicken to a clean cutting board. When cool enough to handle, remove the meat from the bones and shred.
2. Meanwhile, add sweet potato, bell pepper and green beans to the pot; return to a simmer. Cook until the vegetables are tender, 4 to 10 minutes. Stir in the shredded chicken, chickpeas, salt and pepper and cook until heated through, about 3 minutes. Remove from heat.
3. Cover and refrigerate, without the harissa, for up to 3 days. To serve, reheat and then stir in harissa.

Nutritional Value (Amount per Serving):

Calories: 238; Fat: 6.46; Carb: 19.39; Protein: 28.37

Chopped Chicken & Sweet Potato Salad

Prep Time: 10 Minutes   Cook Time: 10 Minutes   Serves: 1

Ingredients:

- 3 cups coarsely chopped escarole or romaine lettuce
- ½ cup cooked diced sweet potato
- 3 ounces shredded cooked chicken
- ¼ cup sliced apple
- 2 tablespoons apple-cider vinaigrette (see Tip)
- ¼ cup chopped avocado
- 2 tablespoons roasted unsalted sunflower seeds
- ½ ounce low-fat Cheddar cheese, cubed

Directions:

1. Toss escarole (or romaine), sweet potato, chicken, and apple with

vinaigrette; place on a 9-inch plate, or divide between containers for storing.
2. Top with avocado, sunflower seeds, and Cheddar.
3. Extra dressing will keep, covered, in the refrigerator for up to 5 days. Bring to room temperature before using.

Nutritional Value (Amount per Serving):

Calories: 872; Fat: 61.47; Carb: 53.51; Protein: 31.9

Boiled Chicken

Prep Time: 10 Minutes   Cook Time: 1 Hour 30 Minutes   Serves: 8

Ingredients:

- 1 (3 pound) whole chicken
- 1 large onion, halved - unpeeled
- 3 carrots, cut into chunks - unpeeled
- 2 stalks celery, cut into chunks
- 1 tablespoon whole peppercorns

Directions:

1. Gather all ingredients.
2. Place chicken in a large pot with onion, carrots, celery, and peppercorns; add water to cover by 1 inch.
3. Cover the pot and bring to a boil; reduce heat to a gentle boil and cook until meat falls off the bone, about 90 minutes.
4. Remove chicken from the pot and let sit until cool enough to handle. Shred or chop meat.
5. Cover and refrigerate for up to 3 days.

Nutritional Value (Amount per Serving):

Calories: 366; Fat: 12.05; Carb: 37.57; Protein: 28.01

Chicken Curry Cup of Noodles

Prep Time: 15 Minutes   Cook Time: 15 Minutes   Serves: 3

Ingredients:

- 3 teaspoons reduced-sodium chicken bouillon paste, divided
- 6 teaspoons red curry paste, divided
- 6 tablespoons coconut milk, divided
- 1 ½ cups frozen stir-fry vegetable mix, divided
- 9 ounces chopped cooked boneless, skinless chicken breast, divided

- 1 ½ cups spiralized zucchini noodles, divided
- 3 teaspoons chopped cilantro, divided
- 3 cups very hot water, divided

Directions:

1. Add 1 teaspoon bouillon paste, 2 teaspoons curry paste and 2 tablespoons coconut milk to each of three 1 1/2-pint canning jars. Layer 1/2 cup vegetables, 3 ounces chicken and 1/2 cup noodles in each jar. Top each with 1 teaspoon cilantro. Cover and refrigerate for up to 3 days.
2. To prepare one jar of noodles: Add 1 cup very hot water to a jar. Cover and shake to combine. Uncover and microwave on High in 1-minute increments until steaming hot, 2 to 3 minutes total. Let stand 5 minutes. Stir before eating.

Nutritional Value (Amount per Serving):

Calories: 436; Fat: 15.51; Carb: 58.99; Protein: 16.55

Sweet & Sour Chicken

Prep Time: 20 Minutes   Cook Time: 20 Minutes   Serves: 4

Ingredients:

- ¼ cup no-salt-added ketchup
- ¼ cup pineapple juice
- 3 tablespoons reduced-sodium soy sauce
- 1 tablespoon rice vinegar
- 2 teaspoons honey
- ¼ teaspoon salt
- ½ teaspoon ground pepper
- 2 tablespoons toasted sesame oil, divided
- 1 pound boneless, skinless chicken breasts, cut into bite-size pieces
- 8 ounces small broccoli florets
- 2 cups chopped red bell pepper
- 1 cup diagonally sliced scallions (1-inch)
- 3 cups cooked brown rice

Directions:

1. Whisk ketchup, pineapple juice, soy sauce, vinegar, honey, salt and pepper in a small bowl.
2. Heat 1 tablespoon oil in a large skillet over high heat. Add chicken and cook, turning occasionally, until browned on all sides, 4 to 5 minutes. Transfer to a plate.
3. Wipe the pan clean; return to high heat and add the remaining 1 tablespoon oil. Add broccoli and bell pepper; cook until charred, about 5

minutes. Add scallions and cook for 1 minute. Return the chicken to the pan and add the ketchup mixture. Cook until bubbly and the sauce coats the chicken.

4. Serve over rice.

Nutritional Value (Amount per Serving):

Calories: 608; Fat: 15.82; Carb: 97.32; Protein: 20.63

Simple Lemon Herb Chicken

Prep Time: 5 Minutes   Cook Time: 10 Minutes   Serves: 2

Ingredients:

- 2 (5 ounce) skinless, boneless chicken breast halves
- 1 medium lemon, juiced, divided
- salt and freshly ground black pepper to taste
- 1 tablespoon olive oil
- 1 pinch dried oregano
- 2 sprigs fresh parsley, chopped, for garnish

Directions:

1. Place chicken in a bowl; pour 1/2 of the lemon juice over chicken and season with salt.
2. Heat olive oil in a medium skillet over medium-low heat. Place chicken into hot oil. Add remaining lemon juice and oregano; season with black pepper. Cook chicken until golden brown and the juices run clear, 5 to 10 minutes per side. An instant-read thermometer inserted into the center should read at least 165 degrees F.
3. Garnish chicken with parsley to serve. Cover and refrigerate for up to 3 days.

Nutritional Value (Amount per Serving):

Calories: 174; Fat: 10.25; Carb: 2.06; Protein: 18.04

Mediterranean Chicken with Eggplant

Prep Time: 50 Minutes   Cook Time: 30 Minutes   Serves: 5

Ingredients:

- 3 eggplants, peeled and cut lengthwise into 1/2 inch thick slices
- 3 tablespoons olive oil
- 6 skinless, boneless chicken breast halves - diced
- 1 onion, diced

- 2 tablespoons tomato paste
- ½ cup water
- 2 teaspoons dried oregano
- salt and pepper to taste

Directions:

1. Place eggplant strips in a big pot of lightly salted water and soak for 30 minutes (this will improve the taste; they will leave a brown color in the pot).
2. Remove eggplant from pot and brush lightly with olive oil. Saute or grill until lightly browned and place in a 9x13 inch baking dish. Set aside.
3. Saute diced chicken and onion in a large skillet over medium heat. Stir in tomato paste and water, cover skillet, reduce heat to low and simmer for 10 minutes.
4. Preheat oven to 400 degrees F.
5. Pour chicken/tomato mixture over eggplant. Season with oregano, salt and pepper and cover with aluminum foil. Bake in the preheated oven for 20 minutes.
6. Cover and refrigerate for up to 3 days.

Nutritional Value (Amount per Serving):

Calories: 499; Fat: 15.91; Carb: 23.73; Protein: 65.19

Chicken Freezer Burritos

Prep Time: 25 Minutes   Cook Time: 5 Minutes   Serves: 4

Ingredients:

- 2 teaspoons extra-virgin olive oil or avocado oil
- ½ cup chopped red onion
- 1 teaspoon minced garlic
- 1 (15 ounce) can low-sodium black beans, rinsed
- ½ cup water
- 1 tablespoon minced chipotle pepper in adobo sauce
- 2 cups shredded cooked chicken
- 2 cups chopped kale
- 1 cup reduced-fat sharp Cheddar cheese
- 2 tablespoons chopped fresh cilantro
- ½ teaspoon grated lime zest (Optional)
- 1 tablespoon fresh lime juice
- ¼ teaspoon salt
- 4 (8 inch) whole-wheat tortillas

Directions:

1. Heat oil in a large nonstick skillet over medium heat. Add onion and garlic; cook, stirring often, until the onion starts to soften, about 2 minutes. Add

beans, water and chipotle; bring to a simmer, mashing slightly with the back of a spatula. Stir in chicken and kale; cook until thickened, 1 to 2 minutes. Remove from heat. Stir in Cheddar, cilantro, lime zest, lime juice and salt.

2. Spread 3/4 cup filling on the bottom third of each tortilla, then roll tightly, burrito-style. Individually wrap the burritos tightly in foil and place in a sealable plastic bag. Freeze for up to 3 months.

3. To reheat one frozen burrito, unwrap and transfer to a microwave-safe plate. Cover with a paper towel and microwave on High until heated through, 2 to 3 minutes.

Nutritional Value (Amount per Serving):

Calories: 503; Fat: 28.94; Carb: 39.12; Protein: 21.84

Asian-Inspired Chicken Lettuce Wraps

Prep Time: 25 Minutes   Cook Time: 15 Minutes   Serves: 4

Ingredients:

- 1 bunch green onions, sliced
- 1 (8 ounce) can water chestnuts, drained and diced
- ¼ cup hoisin sauce
- 2 tablespoons light soy sauce
- 1 tablespoon Sriracha
- ¾ tablespoon rice vinegar
- 1 teaspoon minced fresh ginger
- ½ teaspoon red pepper flakes
- 1 tablespoon olive oil
- 1 cup diced yellow onion
- 1 pound ground chicken
- 3 cloves garlic, minced
- 1 tablespoon sesame oil
- salt and ground black pepper to taste
- 8 leaves Bibb lettuce, or more as needed

Directions:

1. Set 2 to 3 tablespoons green onions aside for garnish. Combine remaining green onions, water chestnuts, hoisin sauce, soy sauce, Sriracha, rice vinegar, ginger, and red pepper flakes in a bowl.

2. Heat oil in a large skillet over medium heat. Add onion and cook until softened, about 5 minutes. Add ground chicken, garlic, and sesame oil. Cook and stir until chicken is crumbly and no longer pink, 5 to 10 minutes.

3. Add hoisin mixture to the skillet and cook until heated through, about 5

minutes. Season with salt and pepper.

4. Fill lettuce leaves with chicken mixture and top with reserved green onions.

Calories: 358; Fat: 19.18; Carb: 25.32; Protein: 23.15

Lemon-Roasted Chicken

Prep Time: 10 Minutes   Cook Time: 45 Minutes   Serves: 6

Ingredients:

- 1 whole chicken, cut into 8 pieces
- 1 onion, cut into wedges
- 1 lemon, sliced
- 8 cloves garlic
- 4 sprigs fresh rosemary
- ¼ cup olive oil
- ½ teaspoon salt
- ½ teaspoon ground black pepper

Directions:

1. Preheat the oven to 450 degrees F.
2. Combine chicken, onion, lemon slices, garlic, and rosemary together in a large bowl. Drizzle olive oil and sprinkle salt and black pepper over the chicken mixture; toss to coat. Spread chicken mixture out in the bottom of a baking dish.
3. Bake in the preheated oven until no longer pink at the bone and the juices run clear, 45 to 50 minutes. An instant-read thermometer inserted into the thickest part of a thigh, near the bone, should read at least 165 degrees F.

Nutritional Value (Amount per Serving):

Calories: 437; Fat: 20.76; Carb: 36.77; Protein: 27.52

Duck Breast with Three Red Fruits

Prep Time: 15 Minutes   Cook Time: 19 Minutes   Serves: 2

Ingredients:

- 1 tablespoon butter
- 3 plums, cut into small pieces
- 1 cup fresh strawberries, hulled and halved
- 1 cup fresh raspberries

- 1 tablespoon honey, or to taste
- 1 cinnamon stick
- 1 large boneless duck breast
- salt and freshly ground black pepper

Directions:

1. Melt butter in a saucepan over medium heat. Add plums, strawberries, raspberries, honey, and cinnamon stick. Stir well and simmer until fruit is soft, about 7 minutes.
2. Score duck breast skin in a diamond pattern. Season with salt and pepper.
3. Heat a skillet over medium heat and cook duck until skin is browned, about 7 minutes. Turn over and cook until duck is medium rare, about 5 minutes more. Slice duck breast in half to check for doneness. Continue cooking, if necessary, until an instant-read thermometer inserted into the center reads at least 165 degrees F and breast is still pink in the center. Slice thinly and serve with the warm sauce ladled over top.

Nutritional Value (Amount per Serving):

Calories: 559; Fat: 21.31; Carb: 61.17; Protein: 33.91

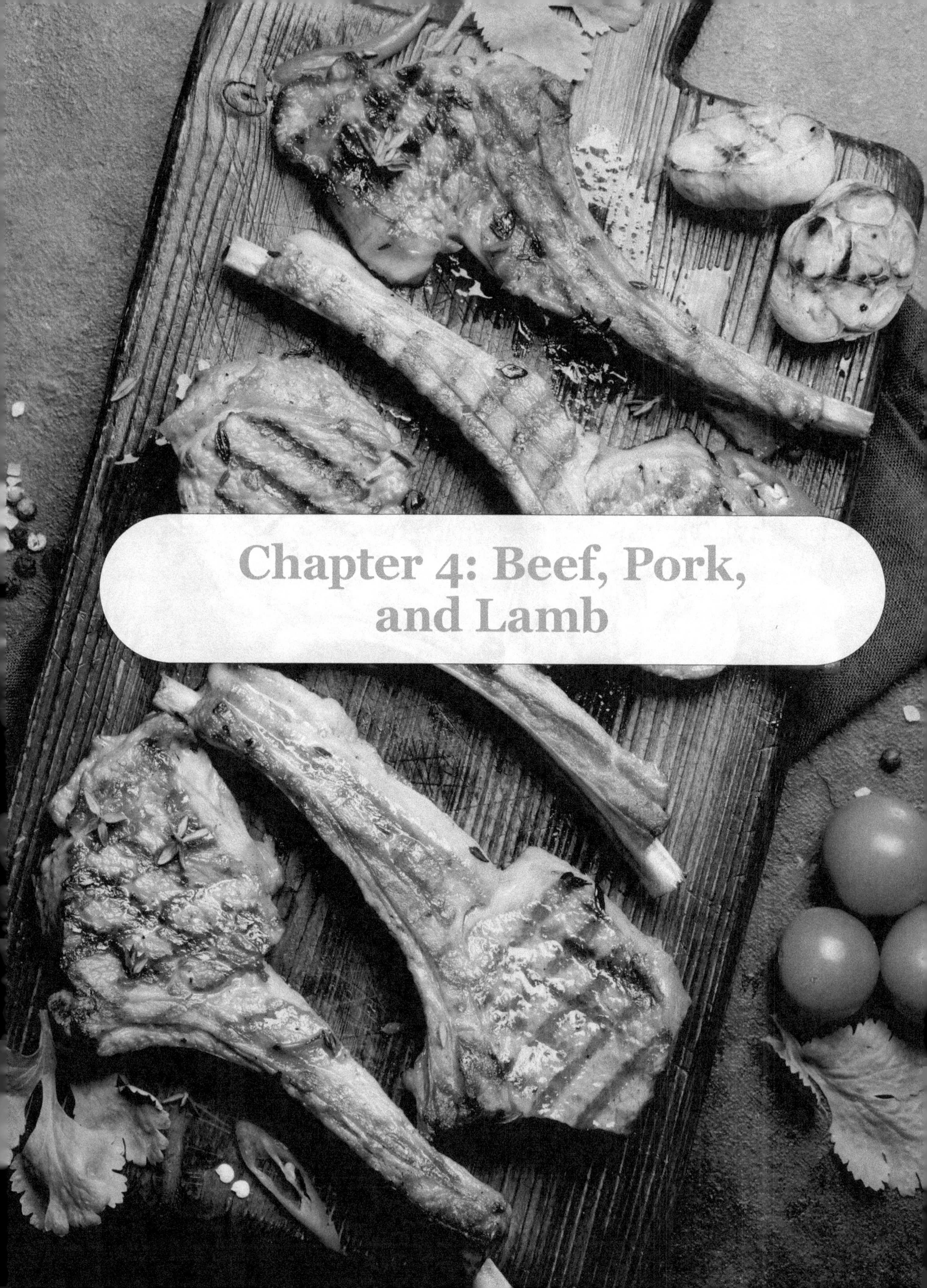
Chapter 4: Beef, Pork, and Lamb

Prep Time: 15 Minutes   Cook Time: 8 Hours   Serves: 8

Ingredients:

- 10 baby red potatoes, quartered
- 4 large carrots, peeled and cut into matchstick pieces
- 1 onion, peeled and cut into bite-sized pieces
- 4 cups water
- 1 (4 pound) corned beef brisket with spice packet
- 6 ounces beer
- ½ head cabbage, coarsely chopped

Directions:

1. Place potatoes, carrots, and onion into the bottom of a slow cooker; add water and place brisket on top of vegetables. Pour beer over brisket; sprinkle over spices from the packet and cover.
2. Cook on High for 7 hours; stir in the cabbage and cook for 1 more hour.
3. Cover and refrigerate for up to 3 days.

Nutritional Value (Amount per Serving):

Calories: 844; Fat: 37.87; Carb: 82.33; Protein: 44.37

Chef John's Perfect Prime Rib

Prep Time: 10 Minutes   Cook Time: 4 Hours 20 Minutes   Serves: 4

Ingredients:

- 1 (4 pound) prime rib roast
- ¼ cup unsalted butter, softened
- 1 tablespoon freshly ground black pepper
- 1 teaspoon herbes de Provence
- kosher salt to taste

Directions:

1. Place prime rib roast on a plate and bring to room temperature, 2 to 4 hours.
2. Preheat the oven to 500 degrees F.
3. Combine butter, pepper, and herbes de Provence in a bowl; mix until well blended. Spread butter mixture evenly over entire roast. Season roast generously with kosher salt.
4. Roast the 4-pound roast in the preheated oven for 20 minutes. (If your roast is larger or smaller than 4 pounds, multiply the exact weight times 5 minutes.)

5. Turn the oven off and, leaving the roast in the oven with the door closed, let the roast sit in the oven for 2 hours.
6. Remove roast from the oven, slice, and refrigerate for up to 3 days.

Calories: 1942; Fat: 167.54; Carb: 0; Protein: 101.58

Instant Pot Corned Beef

Prep Time: 5 Minutes   Cook Time: 1 Hour 55 Minutes   Serves: 4

Ingredients:

- 2 cups water
- 1 (12 fluid ounce) can or bottle beer
- 4 cloves garlic, minced
- 1 (3 pound) corned beef brisket with spice packet

Directions:

1. Gather all ingredients.
2. Combine water, beer, and garlic in a multi-functional pressure cooker.
3. Place trivet inside. Place brisket on the trivet and sprinkle spice packet on top. Close and lock the lid. Select high pressure according to manufacturer's instructions; set timer for 90 minutes. Allow 10 minutes for pressure to build.
4. Release pressure carefully using the quick-release method according to manufacturer's instructions, about 5 minutes. Unlock and remove the lid.
5. Transfer brisket to a baking sheet, cover with aluminum foil, and let rest for 10 to 15 minutes.
6. Cover and refrigerate for up to 2 days.

Nutritional Value (Amount per Serving):

Calories: 687; Fat: 50.7; Carb: 3.76; Protein: 50.13

Jamaican Curried Goat

Prep Time: 15 Minutes   Cook Time: 2 Hours 44 Minutes   Serves: 8

Ingredients:

- 2 pounds goat stew meat, cut into 1-inch cubes
- 2 fresh hot chili peppers, seeded and chopped
- 2 tablespoons curry powder
- 2 cloves garlic, minced
- 1 teaspoon salt

- 1 teaspoon ground black pepper
- 3 tablespoons vegetable oil
- 1 onion, chopped
- 1 rib celery, chopped
- 2 ½ cups vegetable broth
- 1 bay leaf
- 3 potatoes, peeled and cut into 1-inch chunks, or more as desired

Directions:

1. Combine goat meat, chili pepper, curry powder, garlic, salt, and black pepper in a bowl. Cover and refrigerate to allow flavors to blend, 1 hour to overnight.
2. Remove goat meat mixture from bowl and pat dry, reserving marinade. Heat vegetable oil in a stockpot over medium-high heat. Cook meat in batches, browning on all sides, 5 to 6 minutes per batch. Transfer meat to a plate. Add onion and celery to the stockpot; cook and stir until onion begins to brown, 4 to 6 minutes.
3. Stir browned goat meat into onion mixture. Add reserved marinade, vegetable broth, and bay leaf. Bring to a boil, cover, reduce heat to low, and simmer for 1 hour. Stir in potatoes; simmer until potatoes and meat are tender, 35 to 45 minutes.
4. Remove stockpot from heat, skim off surface fat, and remove bay leaf. Cool it, divide into different containers and refrigerate for up to 2 days.

Nutritional Value (Amount per Serving):

Calories: 339; Fat: 12.69; Carb: 28.64; Protein: 27.57

Roasted Rack of Lamb

Prep Time: 15 Minutes   Cook Time: 30 Minutes   Serves: 4

Ingredients:

- ½ cup fresh bread crumbs
- 2 tablespoons minced garlic
- 2 tablespoons chopped fresh rosemary
- 1 teaspoon salt
- ¼ teaspoon black pepper
- 2 tablespoons olive oil
- 1 (7 bone) rack of lamb, trimmed and frenched
- 1 teaspoon salt
- 1 teaspoon black pepper
- 2 tablespoons olive oil
- 1 tablespoon Dijon mustard

1. Preheat the oven to 450 degrees F. Move the oven rack to the center position.
2. Combine bread crumbs, garlic, rosemary, 1 teaspoon salt, and 1/4 teaspoon pepper in a small bowl; stir in 2 tablespoons olive oil to moisten the mixture. Set aside.
3. Season rack of lamb all over with 1 teaspoon salt and 1 teaspoon pepper. Heat 2 tablespoons olive oil in a large heavy oven-proof skillet over high heat. Add lamb and sear on all sides, about 1 to 2 minutes: set lamb aside for a few minutes. Brush lamb with mustard and roll in bread crumb mixture until evenly coated. Cover the ends of the bones with foil to prevent charring.
4. Arrange the breaded rack of lamb bone-side down in the same skillet. Roast in preheated oven for 12 to 18 minutes for medium; an instant-read thermometer inserted into the center should read at least 130 degrees F, or continue to cook to desired doneness. Remove lamb from the skillet and allow to rest for 5 to 7 minutes, loosely covered with foil, before carving between the ribs.
5. Refrigerate for up to 2 days or freeze for up to 1 month.

Nutritional Value (Amount per Serving):

Calories: 543; Fat: 35.4; Carb: 4.55; Protein: 52.55

Roasted Lamb Breast

Prep Time: 30 Minutes   Cook Time: 2 Hours 25 Minutes   Serves: 4

Ingredients:

- 2 tablespoons olive oil
- 2 teaspoons ground cumin
- 2 teaspoons salt
- 1 teaspoon freshly ground black pepper
- 1 teaspoon dried Italian herb seasoning
- 1 teaspoon ground cinnamon
- 1 teaspoon ground coriander
- 1 teaspoon paprika
- 4 pounds lamb breast, separated in two pieces
- aluminum foil
- ½ cup chopped Italian flat leaf parsley
- ⅓ cup white wine vinegar, more as needed
- 1 lemon, juiced
- 2 cloves garlic, crushed

- 1 teaspoon honey
- ½ teaspoon red pepper flakes
- 1 pinch salt

Directions:

1. Preheat the oven to 300 degrees F.
2. Whisk olive oil, cumin, salt, black pepper, Italian herb seasoning, cinnamon, coriander, and paprika in a large bowl until combined.
3. Coat lamb breasts in spice mixture, then place fat-side-up in a roasting pan. Tightly cover the roasting pan with aluminum foil.
4. Bake in the preheated oven until meat is tender when pierced with a fork, about 2 hours.
5. Meanwhile, combine chopped parsley, vinegar, fresh lemon juice, garlic, honey, red pepper flakes, and salt in a bowl. Mix well and set aside.
6. Remove meat from the oven.
7. Increase oven temperature to 450 degrees F. Line a baking sheet with aluminum foil.
8. Remove lamb from the roasting pan and cut into 4 pieces. Place lamb pieces on the prepared baking sheet. Brush tops with fat drippings from the roasting pan.
9. Roast in the preheated oven until meat is browned and edges are crispy, about 20 minutes.
10. Turn the oven broiler to high and brown meat until top is golden brown, about 4 minutes.
11. Refrigerate for up to 2 days.
12. Serve lamb topped with parsley-vinegar sauce.

Nutritional Value (Amount per Serving):

Calories: 780; Fat: 44.45; Carb: 12.27; Protein: 84.56

Grilled Lamb Loin Chops

Prep Time: 5 Minutes   Cook Time: 1 Hour 15 Minutes   Serves: 4

Ingredients:

- 2 tablespoons herbes de Provence
- 1 ½ tablespoons olive oil
- 2 cloves garlic, minced
- 2 teaspoons lemon juice
- 8 (5 ounce) lamb loin chops
- salt and ground black pepper to taste

Directions:

1. Combine herbes de Provence, oil, garlic, and lemon juice in a small bowl. Rub mixture over lamb chops; cover and refrigerate for at least 1 hour, or up to 4 hours for maximum flavor.

2. Preheat an outdoor grill for medium-high heat and lightly oil the grate.
3. Season chops with salt and pepper.
4. Place chops on the preheated grill, and cook until browned on the outside and an instant-read thermometer inserted into the center reads at least 125 degrees F for medium-rare, 3 to 4 minutes per side.
5. Transfer chops to an aluminum foil-covered plate; let cool before storing in refrigerator.

Nutritional Value (Amount per Serving):

Calories: 103; Fat: 7.55; Carb: 1.75; Protein: 7.41

Burgundy Pork Tenderloin

Prep Time: 30 Minutes   Cook Time: 1 Hour   Serves: 4

Ingredients:

- 2 pounds pork tenderloin
- ½ teaspoon salt
- ½ teaspoon ground black pepper
- ½ teaspoon garlic powder
- ½ onion, thinly sliced
- 1 stalk celery, chopped
- 2 cups red wine
- 1 (.75 ounce) packet dry brown gravy mix

Directions:

1. Preheat oven to 350 degrees F.
2. Place pork in a 9x13 inch baking dish, and sprinkle meat with salt, pepper and garlic powder. Top with onion and celery, and pour wine all over.
3. Bake in the preheated oven for 45 minutes.
4. When done baking, remove meat from baking dish, and place on a serving platter. Pour gravy mix into baking dish with wine and cooking juices, and stir until thickened.
5. Slice meat, and cover in refrigerator for up to 2 days. And serve with the gravy.

Nutritional Value (Amount per Serving):

Calories: 1351; Fat: 7.98; Carb: 300.6; Protein: 59.62

Italian Pork Tenderloin

Prep Time: 15 Minutes   Cook Time: 35 Minutes   Serves: 4

- 2 tablespoons olive oil
- ¼ cup chopped prosciutto
- 2 tablespoons chopped fresh sage
- 2 tablespoons chopped fresh parsley
- 2 tablespoons chopped oil-packed sun-dried tomatoes
- ¼ cup chopped onion
- 1 ½ pounds pork tenderloin, cut into 1/2 inch strips
- ½ cup chicken broth
- ½ cup heavy cream
- ¼ teaspoon salt
- ½ teaspoon ground black pepper

Directions:

1. Heat the oil in a skillet over medium-high heat. Saute the prosciutto, sage, parsley, sun-dried tomatoes, and onion 5 minutes, until onion is tender. Mix the pork strips into the skillet, and brown about 10 minutes, turning once.
2. Stir the broth and heavy cream into the skillet, and season with salt and pepper. Bring to a boil. Reduce heat to low, and simmer 20 minutes, stirring occasionally, until pork reaches a minimum temperature of 145 degrees F and sauce is thickened.
3. Refrigerate for up to 2 days.

Nutritional Value (Amount per Serving):

Calories: 439; Fat: 22.08; Carb: 3.39; Protein: 54.35

Charcoal-Grilled Ribeye Steak

Prep Time: 5 Minutes   Cook Time: 6 Minutes   Serves: 1

Ingredients:

- 1 (12 ounce) ribeye steak
- 1/2 teaspoon seasoned salt, such as Lawry's Seasoned Salt
- 1/4 teaspoon freshly cracked black pepper, or to taste

Directions:

1. Season steak evenly, using 1/4 teaspoon seasoned salt and 1/8 teaspoon black pepper on each side. Set aside.
2. Light charcoal briquettes. Once they are red hot, place steak on the grates. Grill for 4 to 5 minutes. Turn steak over and grill an additional 2 to 3 minutes.
3. Tent steak with aluminum foil and let rest 4 to 5 minutes before serving.

Nutritional Value (Amount per Serving):

Calories: 470; Fat: 28.41; Carb: 5.43; Protein: 48.68

Air Fryer New York Strip Steak

Prep Time: 5 Minutes   Cook Time: 10 Minutes   Serves: 3

Ingredients:

- 3 New York strip steaks, about 1 1/4-inch thick
- 1/2 teaspoon your favorite seasoned salt, or to taste
- 1/2 teaspoon Montreal steak seasoning, or other seasoning of choice
- olive oil cooking spray
- 1 teaspoon Worcestershire sauce, or to taste (optional)

Directions:

1. About 30 minutes before cooking, remove the steaks from the refrigerator and allow them to come to room temperature. Pat steaks dry with paper towels, and sprinkle seasoning salt and Montreal Steak Seasoning on both sides.
2. Preheat the air fryer to 400 degrees F, according to manufacturer's instructions.
3. When the air fryer is fully preheated, spray both sides of steaks with olive oil cooking spray.
4. Place steaks in the air fryer and cook about 10 minutes for medium rare, turning halfway through.
5. Check the temperature of the meat before removing from the air fryer. For medium-rare, an instant-read thermometer inserted into the center should read 130 degrees F. Tent with foil, about 10 minutes. Serve warm.

Nutritional Value (Amount per Serving):

Calories: 254; Fat: 5.84; Carb: 0.66; Protein: 49.39

Ultimate Tomahawk Steak

Prep Time: 5 Minutes   Cook Time: 30 Minutes   Serves: 4

Ingredients:

- 3 1/2 pound tomahawk rib eye steak
- 1 1/2 tablespoons kosher salt
- 2 1/2 teaspoons ground black pepper

Directions:

1. Remove steak from refrigerator and let stand at room temperature 30 minutes to an hour before cooking.

2. Preheat the grill to medium-high, 400 to 450 degrees F. Sprinkle steak evenly and liberally on all sides with salt and black pepper.
3. Lightly coat grill grates with oil or grilling spray. Place steak on hot grates, and grill, undisturbed, until it releases easily from the grates, about 4 minutes. Flip, and repeat on the other side. Continue grilling, turning occasionally, until a thermometer inserted into the thickest portion of steak registers 125 degrees F, 30 to 40 minutes.
4. Transfer steak to a cutting board; let rest 15 minutes. Run a knife along the inside edge of the bone to remove steak from the bone in 1 piece; slice against the grain to serve.

Nutritional Value (Amount per Serving):

Calories: 1043; Fat: 83.25; Carb: 2.66; Protein: 71.69

The Best Easy Pork Tenderloin

Prep Time: 5 Minutes   Cook Time: 30 Minutes   Serves: 8

Ingredients:

- 2 pork tenderloins (1 lb. each)
- 1 1/2 teaspoons salt
- 1 teaspoon freshly ground black pepper
- 1 teaspoon granulated garlic
- 2 teaspoon herbes de Provence
- 4 teaspoons olive oil
- 1/2 cup white wine or chicken stock

Directions:

1. Preheat the oven to 400 degrees F. Trim the silver skin from each pork tenderloin and season evenly with salt, pepper, garlic, and herbes de Provence.
2. Heat oil in a large oven-proof skillet over medium-high heat until barely shimmering. Add both pork tenderloins and cook, undisturbed, until golden brown and easily release from the pan, about 5 minutes. Flip each piece and cook for an additional 3 minutes undisturbed. Add wine and cook for 1 minute. Remove pan from the stove and place in the oven.
3. Bake in the preheated oven until pork is slightly pink in the center, 15 to 19 minutes. An instant-read thermometer inserted into the center should read at least 145 degrees F.
4. Remove from the oven and allow to rest for 5 to 10 minutes before slicing. Serve with pan juices.

Nutritional Value (Amount per Serving):

Calories: 195; Fat: 7.01; Carb: 0.28; Protein: 30.73

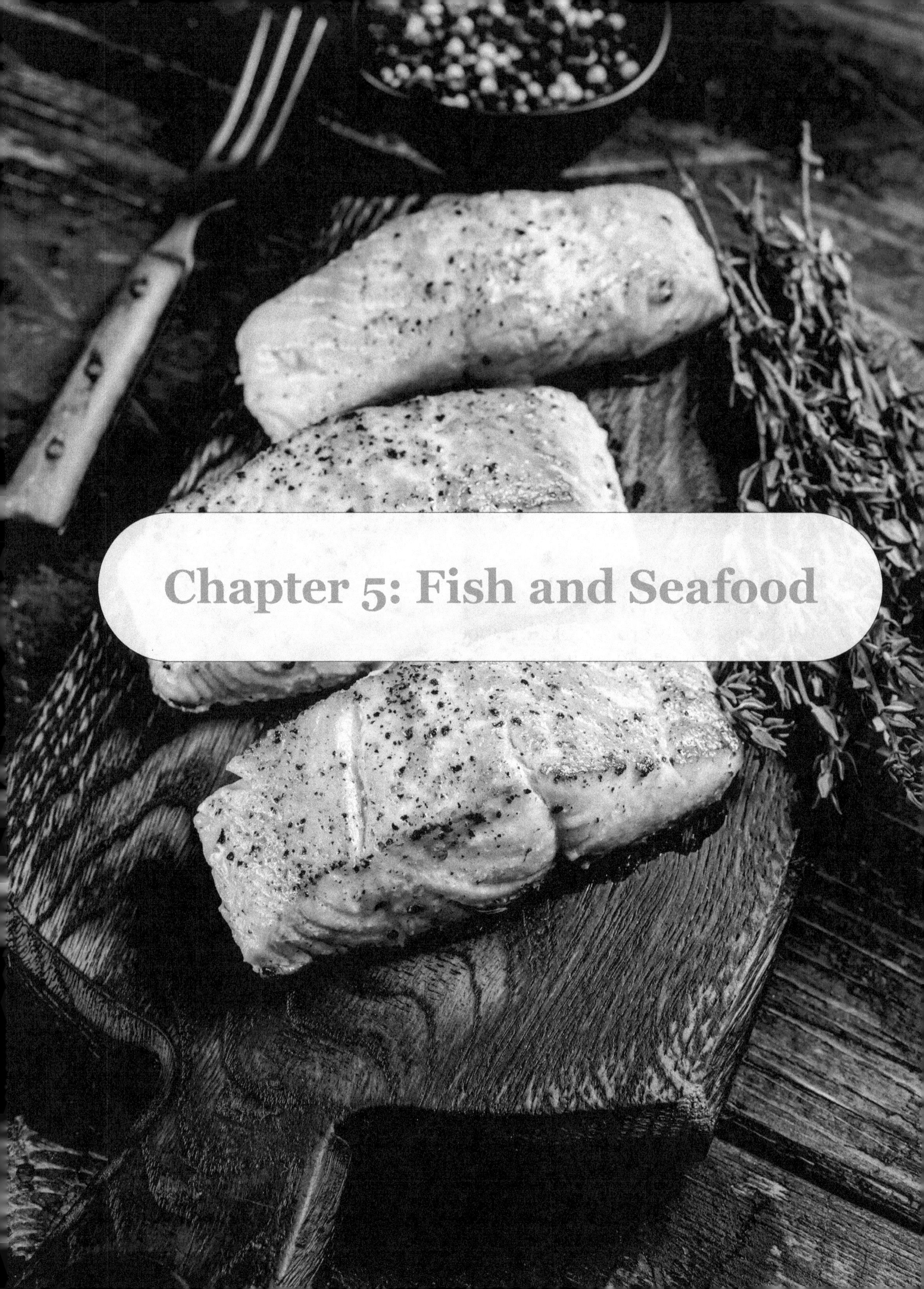
Chapter 5: Fish and Seafood

Kimchi Shrimp Cup of Noodles

Prep Time: 15 Minutes   Cook Time: 15 Minutes   Serves: 3

Ingredients:

- 3 teaspoons reduced-sodium chicken bouillon paste, divided
- 3 teaspoons gochujang, divided
- 1 ½ cups chopped cabbage, divided
- 1 ½ cups sliced mushrooms, divided
- ¾ cup chopped kimchi, divided
- 9 ounces cooked shrimp, divided
- 1 ½ cups cooked rice noodles, divided
- 1 sliced radish, divided
- 2 teaspoons chopped cilantro, divided
- 3 slices lime, divided
- 3 cups very hot water, divided

Directions:

1. Place 1 teaspoon bouillon paste and 1 teaspoon gochujang in each of three 1 1/2-pint canning jars. Layer 1/2 cup cabbage, 1/2 cup mushrooms, 1/4 cup kimchi, 3 ounces shrimp and 1/2 cup noodles in each jar. Top each with some radish slices, 1 teaspoon cilantro and 1 lime slice. Cover and refrigerate for up to 3 days.
2. To prepare one jar of noodles: Add 1 cup very hot water to a jar. Cover and shake to combine. Uncover and microwave on High in 1-minute increments until steaming hot, 2 to 3 minutes total. Let stand 5 minutes. Stir before eating.

Nutritional Value (Amount per Serving):

Calories: 245; Fat: 4.27; Carb: 30.46; Protein: 21.86

Mason Jar Power Salad with Chickpeas & Tuna

Prep Time: 5 Minutes   Cook Time: 5 Minutes   Serves: 4

Ingredients:

- 3 cups bite-sized pieces chopped kale
- 2 tablespoons honey-mustard vinaigrette (see associated recipe)
- 1 2.5-ounce pouch tuna in water
- ½ cup rinsed canned chickpeas
- 1 carrot, peeled and shredded

Directions:

1. Toss kale and dressing in a bowl, then transfer to a 1-quart mason jar. Top

with tuna, chickpeas and carrot. Screw lid onto the jar and refrigerate for up to 2 days.
   2. To serve, empty the jar contents into a bowl, and toss to combine the salad ingredients with the dressed kale.

Nutritional Value (Amount per Serving):

Calories: 141; Fat: 4.72; Carb: 20; Protein: 5.84

Tuna Salad Crackers

Prep Time: 5 Minutes   Cook Time: 5 Minutes   Serves: 1

Ingredients:

- 6 wheat crackers
- 1 2.6-ounce pouch low-sodium light tuna
- 1 tablespoon reduced-fat olive oil mayonnaise
- ½ cup red pepper strips
- ½ cup cucumber slices
- 1 single-serve sun-dried-tomato hummus dip

Directions:

1. Mix tuna and mayonnaise. Spread on crackers. Serve with peppers, cucumbers, and hummus.
2. Tuna mix can be refrigerate for up to 2 days.

Nutritional Value (Amount per Serving):

Calories: 364; Fat: 16.85; Carb: 27.6; Protein: 27.93

Pan-Seared Salmon

Prep Time: 10 Minutes   Cook Time: 10 Minutes   Serves: 4

Ingredients:

- 4 (6 ounce) fillets salmon
- 2 tablespoons olive oil
- 2 tablespoons capers
- ⅛ teaspoon salt
- ⅛ teaspoon ground black pepper
- 4 slices lemon

Directions:

1. Preheat a large heavy skillet over medium heat for 3 minutes.
2. Coat salmon fillets with olive oil; place skin-side down in the preheated skillet and increase heat to high.
3. Sprinkle with capers, salt, and pepper; cook for 3 minutes on one side. Turn salmon fillets over; continue to cook until salmon flakes easily with a fork, about 5 minutes.

4. Transfer salmon to individual plates and garnish with lemon slices.
5. Or refrigerate for up to 2 days.

Nutritional Value (Amount per Serving):

Calories: 137; Fat: 9.95; Carb: 3.66; Protein: 9.07

Baked Asian Rockfish

Prep Time: 10 Minutes   Cook Time: 10 Minutes   Serves: 4

Ingredients:

- 4 (6 ounce) rockfish filets
- 1 tablespoon sesame oil
- 2 cloves garlic, minced
- 1 tablespoon finely minced fresh ginger
- 1 tablespoon honey
- 1/4 teaspoon red pepper flakes
- 1 tablespoon soy sauce
- 1 tablespoon lime juice
- 1/4 cup diagonally thinly sliced scallions

Directions:

1. Preheat the oven to 400 degrees F. Line a shallow baking pan with aluminum foil, and spray with cooking spray. Place filets onto the prepared baking pan.
2. In a small bowl combine sesame oil, soy sauce, lime juice, honey, ginger, garlic, and pepper flakes. Spoon mixture evenly over top of filets.
3. Bake in the preheated oven until fish flakes easily with a fork, 10 to 15 minutes.
4. Or refrigerate for up to 2 days. Sprinkle filets with scallions before serving.

Nutritional Value (Amount per Serving):

Calories: 121; Fat: 6.41; Carb: 6.66; Protein: 9.33

Salmon Couscous Salad

Prep Time: 10 Minutes   Cook Time: 10 Minutes   Serves: 1

Ingredients:

- ¼ cup sliced cremini mushrooms
- ¼ cup diced eggplant
- 3 cups baby spinach
- 2 tablespoons white-wine vinaigrette, divided (see Tip)

- ¼ cup cooked Israeli couscous, preferably whole-wheat
- 4 ounces cooked salmon
- ¼ cup sliced dried apricots
- 2 tablespoons crumbled goat cheese (1/2 ounce)

Directions:

1. Coat a small skillet with cooking spray and heat over medium-high heat. Add mushrooms and eggplant; cook, stirring, until lightly browned and juices have been released, 3 to 5 minutes. Remove from heat and set aside.
2. Toss spinach with 1 Tbsp. plus 1 tsp. vinaigrette, and place on a 9-inch plate.
3. Toss couscous with the remaining 2 tsp. vinaigrette and place on top of the spinach. Place salmon on top. Top with the cooked vegetables, dried apricots, and goat cheese.
4. Extra will keep, covered, in the refrigerator for up to 5 days.
5. Bring to room temperature before eating.

Nutritional Value (Amount per Serving):

Calories: 387; Fat: 13.93; Carb: 34.8; Protein: 33.66

Baked Whole Crappie

Prep Time: 25 Minutes   Cook Time: 20 Minutes   Serves: 4

Ingredients:

- 4 whole crappie fish, gutted and cleaned, tails still on
- 1 bunch fresh cilantro
- 1/4 cup extra virgin olive oil
- 2 tablespoons lime juice
- 3 cloves garlic
- 2 teaspoons salt
- 1 teaspoon paprika
- 8 thin lemon slices

Directions:

1. Preheat the oven to 400 degrees F. Line a shallow baking pan with aluminum foil.
2. Pat fish dry; score the skin of fish in a diamond pattern with a very sharp knife. Place fish on the prepared baking pan. Cover tails of fish with aluminum foil to avoid overbrowning.
3. Combine cilantro, olive oil, lime juice, garlic, salt, and paprika in a blender; pulse until mixture is a soft paste.
4. Spread cilantro-garlic paste on each fish, pressing the paste into the scored sections. Place 2 lemon slices on each fish.

5. Bake, uncovered, in the preheated oven until fish flakes easily when tested with a fork, about 20 minutes.
6. Keep in the refrigerator for up to 2 days.

Calories: 1310; Fat: 77.15; Carb: 8.33; Protein: 139.25

Pan-Seared Red Snapper

Prep Time: 10 Minutes   Cook Time: 10 Minutes   Serves: 2

Ingredients:

- ¼ cup chopped green onions
- 1 lemon, juiced
- 2 tablespoons rice wine vinegar
- 1 tablespoon olive oil
- 1 tablespoon honey
- 1 teaspoon Dijon mustard
- 1 teaspoon ground ginger
- 2 (4 ounce) fillets red snapper

Directions:

1. Gather all ingredients.
2. Mix together green onions, lemon juice, vinegar, olive oil, honey, mustard, and ginger in a shallow bowl; set aside.
3. Rinse snapper under cold water and pat dry with paper towels.
4. Heat a large nonstick skillet over medium heat. Dip snapper into marinade to coat both sides.
5. Cook snapper in the hot skillet until opaque and lightly browned, 2 to 3 minutes per side.
6. Pour remaining marinade into the skillet. Reduce heat and simmer until fish flakes easily with a fork, 2 to 3 minutes.
7. Keep in the refrigerator for up to 3 days.

Nutritional Value (Amount per Serving):

Calories: 159; Fat: 7.04; Carb: 24.99; Protein: 0.85

Spicy Slaw Bowls with Shrimp & Edamame

Prep Time: 15 Minutes   Cook Time: 15 Minutes   Serves:4

Ingredients:

- Spicy Cabbage Slaw
- 2 cups frozen shelled edamame, thawed
- 1 medium avocado, diced
- ½ medium lime, juiced
- 12 ounces peeled cooked shrimp

Directions:

1. Prepare Spicy Cabbage Slaw. Add edamame; toss and set aside.
2. Toss avocado with lime juice in a small bowl.
3. Divide the slaw mixture among 4 containers. Top each with 1/4 of the shrimp (about 3 ounces) and 1/4 of the avocado.
4. Cover and refrigerate until ready to eat.

Nutritional Value (Amount per Serving):

Calories: 268; Fat: 12.59; Carb: 14.09; Protein: 27.15

Firecracker Salmon

Prep Time: 10 Minutes   Cook Time: 45 Minutes   Serves: 2

Ingredients:

- ¼ cup maple syrup
- 1 medium jalapeño, cut in half width-wise
- 1 clove garlic, minced
- 1 tablespoon rice wine vinegar
- ½ teaspoon salt
- ⅛ teaspoon black pepper
- 2 (6 ounce) fillets salmon fillets
- salt and pepper to taste
- 2 teaspoons maple syrup

Directions:

1. Combine 1/4 cup maple syrup, 1/2 of the jalapeño pepper, garlic, vinegar, salt, and black pepper in a mini food processor or small blender jar; blend until smooth.
2. Place salmon fillets in a gallon-sized resealable plastic bag. Pour marinade on top, seal, and refrigerate for 20 minutes. Remove from refrigerator and let the bag sit at room temperature for 10 minutes.
3. Preheat the oven to 425 degrees F. Line a baking sheet with parchment paper.
4. Remove salmon from marinade and pat dry. Place salmon on the prepared baking sheet and season with additional salt and pepper. Slice remaining jalapeno pepper thinly and place on top of salmon.
5. Bake in the preheated oven for 10 minutes. Brush 2 teaspoons maple syrup onto the fillets and return to the hot oven. Bake until fish flakes easily with a fork, an additional 3 to 5 minutes.

Nutritional Value (Amount per Serving):

Calories: 268; Fat: 6.26; Carb: 34.56; Protein: 18.27

Fast Salmon with a Ginger Glaze

Prep Time: 5 Minutes   Cook Time: 20 Minutes   Serves: 4

Ingredients:

- 4 (8 ounce) fresh salmon fillets
- salt to taste
- ⅓ cup cold water
- ¼ cup seasoned rice vinegar
- 2 tablespoons brown sugar
- 1 tablespoon hot chile paste (such as sambal oelek)
- 1 tablespoon finely grated fresh ginger
- 4 cloves garlic, minced
- 1 teaspoon soy sauce
- ¼ cup chopped fresh basil

Directions:

1. Preheat grill for medium heat and lightly oil the grate.
2. Season salmon fillets with salt.
3. Place salmon on the preheated grill; cook salmon for 6 to 8 minutes per side, or until the fish flakes easily with a fork.
4. Combine water, rice vinegar, brown sugar, chile paste, ginger, garlic, and soy sauce in a small saucepan over medium heat.
5. Bring mixture to a boil, reduce heat to medium and simmer until barely thickened, about 2 minutes.
6. Sprinkle basil on top of salmon; spoon glaze over basil.

Nutritional Value (Amount per Serving):

Calories: 110; Fat: 4.35; Carb: 4.45; Protein: 12.08

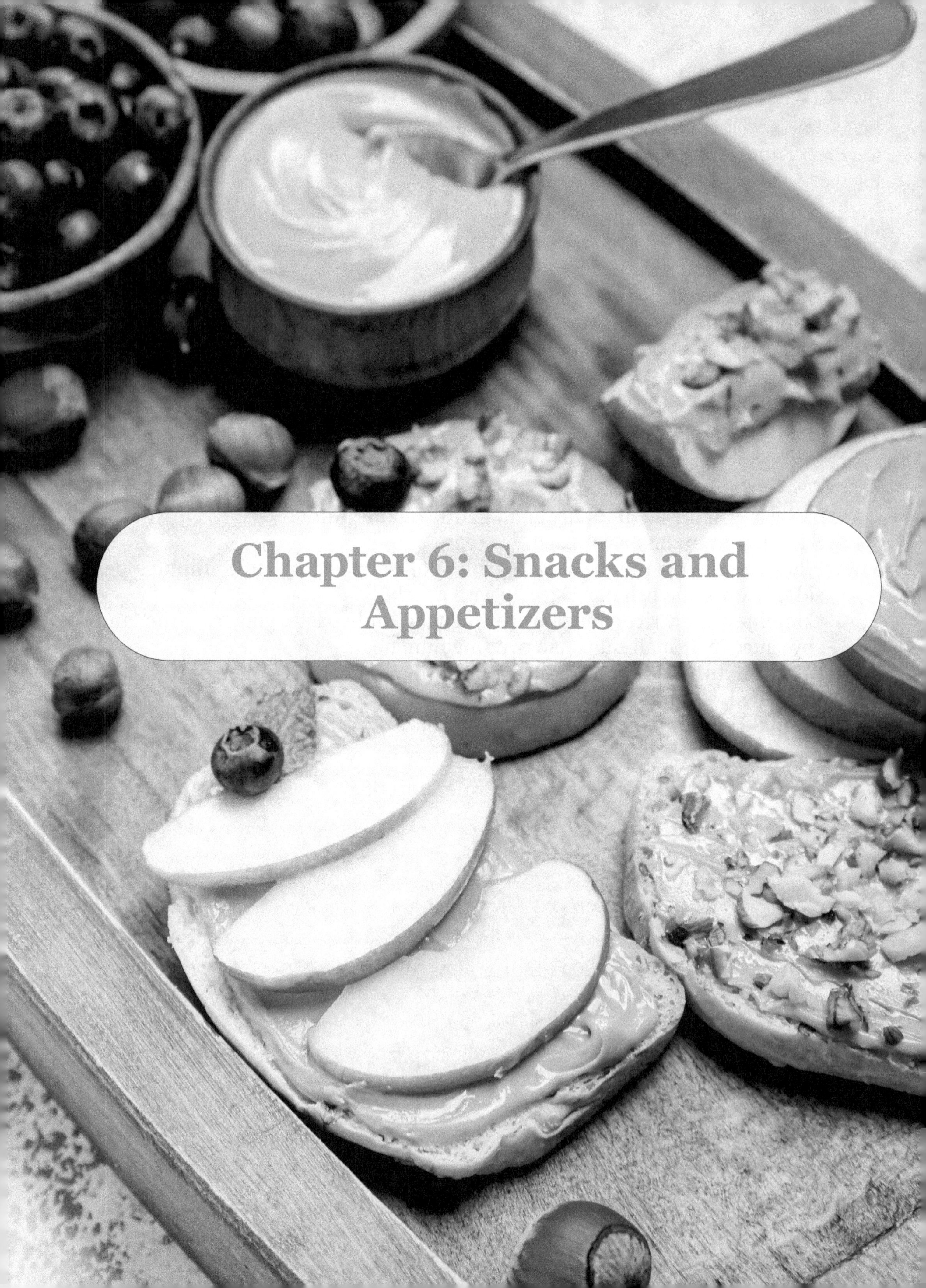

Chapter 6: Snacks and Appetizers

Clean-Eating Bento Box

Prep Time: 10 Minutes   Cook Time: 10 Minutes   Serves:1

Ingredients:

- ½ cup snap peas
- ¼ cup blueberries
- ½ medium apple, sliced
- 8 seeded whole-grain crackers, such as Mary's Gone Crackers
- 1 ounce Cheddar cheese, sliced
- 2 tablespoons hummus

Directions:

1. Pack snap peas, blueberries, apple, cheese, hummus and crackers in a divided bento-style lunch box or in separate containers with lids.
2. Refrigerate for up to 1 day.

Nutritional Value (Amount per Serving):

Calories: 1142; Fat: 41.82; Carb: 165.83; Protein: 27.78

Easy Garlic Escargots

Prep Time: 15 Minutes   Cook Time: 30 Minutes   Serves: 4

Ingredients:

- 1 (7 ounce) can escargots, drained
- 6 tablespoons butter
- 1 clove garlic, minced
- 20 mushrooms, stems removed
- ⅓ cup white wine
- ⅓ cup cream
- 1 tablespoon all-purpose flour
- ¼ teaspoon dried tarragon
- 1 pinch freshly ground black pepper, or to taste
- ¼ cup grated Parmesan cheese

Directions:

1. Place escargots in a small bowl and cover with cold water. Let sit for 5 minutes to remove any canned flavor they may have.
2. Preheat the oven to 350 degrees F. Lightly grease an 8x8-inch baking dish.
3. Drain escargots and pat dry with a paper towel.
4. Melt butter with garlic in a large skillet over medium-high heat. Add escargots and mushroom caps; cook and stir until mushroom caps begin to soften, about 5 minutes.
5. Whisk together wine, cream, flour, tarragon, and pepper in a small bowl until well combined. Pour into the skillet and bring to a boil. Cook, stirring

occasionally, until sauce thickens, about 10 minutes. Remove from the heat.

6. Place mushroom caps into the prepared baking dish, with the tops facing down. Spoon an escargot into each mushroom cap. Pour sauce from the skillet over mushroom caps, then sprinkle grated Parmesan cheese over top.
7. Bake in the preheated oven until cheese has turned golden brown, 10 to 15 minutes.
8. Cover and refrigerate until ready to eat.

Calories: 304; Fat: 24.45; Carb: 17.73; Protein: 7.68

Roasted Pumpkin Seeds

Prep Time: 5 Minutes   Cook Time: 45 Minutes   Serves: 6

Ingredients:

- 1 ½ cups raw whole pumpkin seeds
- 1 pinch salt
- 2 teaspoons butter, melted

Directions:

1. Preheat oven to 300 degrees F and gather ingredients.
2. Toss seeds in a bowl with the melted butter and salt. Spread the seeds in a single layer on a baking sheet and bake for about 45 minutes or until golden brown; stir occasionally.
3. Store in room temperature.

Calories: 83; Fat: 4.39; Carb: 8.6; Protein: 2.98

Best-Ever Texas Caviar

Prep Time: 25 Minutes   Cook Time: 15 Minutes   Serves: 10

Ingredients:

- 2 (15 ounce) cans black beans, rinsed and drained
- 2 (15 ounce) cans pinto beans, rinsed and drained
- 2 (15 ounce) cans white corn, rinsed and drained
- 1 (4 ounce) can chopped green chilies, undrained
- 1 red bell pepper - cored, seeded and finely chopped
- 1 green bell pepper - cored, seeded and finely chopped
- 1 small red onion, finely chopped

- 1 jalapeno chili pepper, seeded and finely chopped (Optional)
- 1 bunch cilantro leaves, finely chopped
- ½ cup rice vinegar
- ½ cup olive oil
- ⅓ cup white sugar
- ½ teaspoon garlic powder

Directions:

1. Gather all ingredients.
2. Mix together black beans, pinto beans, white corn, green chilies, red and green bell peppers, red onion, jalapeño pepper, and cilantro in a large bowl.
3. Combine rice vinegar, olive oil, sugar, and garlic powder in a pan. Bring to a boil, then remove from heat. Let cool for at least 10 minutes. Cover and refrigerate until ready to eat.
4. When ready to eat, pour dressing over bean mixture; toss to coat.

Nutritional Value (Amount per Serving):

Calories: 370; Fat: 14.06; Carb: 49.27; Protein: 14.94

Grilled Halloumi with Herbed Berry Salsa

Prep Time: 20 Minutes   Cook Time: 15 Minutes   Serves: 4

Ingredients:

- 4 ounces fresh blueberries
- 3 ounces red currants
- 3 tablespoons chopped fresh mint, divided
- 3 tablespoons chopped fresh cilantro, divided
- 1 tablespoon fresh marjoram, stems removed
- 1 habanero pepper, seeded and minced
- 2 tablespoons olive oil
- 2 tablespoons agave syrup
- 2 limes, divided
- ½ cup cashews
- 8 ounces halloumi cheese, cut into 8 slices

Directions:

1. Place blueberries and red currants into a mixing bowl. Add 2 tablespoons mint, 2 tablespoons cilantro, marjoram, habanero, olive oil, agave syrup, and juice of 1 lime. Mix and set aside.
2. Heat a nonstick griddle over medium-high heat. Cook cashews until browned, stirring often to keep from burning, 8 to 10 minutes. Transfer cashews to a plate and set aside. Reduce heat to medium and brown

halloumi cheese slices, 2 to 3 minutes per side.

3. Place halloumi cheese onto a plate, top with berry salsa mixture and remaining 1 tablespoon mint and cilantro. Chop cashews and spread on top of halloumi. Garnish with lime wedges from remaining lime.
4. Cover and refrigerate until ready to eat.

Nutritional Value (Amount per Serving):

Calories: 803; Fat: 56.16; Carb: 28.55; Protein: 48.66

Mango Salsa

Prep Time: 15 Minutes   Cook Time: 30 Minutes   Serves: 8

Ingredients:

- 1 mango - peeled, seeded, and chopped
- ¼ cup finely chopped red bell pepper
- 1 green onion, chopped
- 1 fresh jalapeño chili pepper, finely chopped
- 2 tablespoons chopped cilantro
- 2 tablespoons lime juice
- 1 tablespoon lemon juice

Directions:

1. Gather ingredients.
2. Place mango, red bell pepper, green onion, jalapeño, cilantro, lime juice, and lemon juice in a medium bowl.
3. Mix ingredients well to combine. Cover and let sit at least 30 minutes before serving.
4. Serve with chips.

Nutritional Value (Amount per Serving):

Calories: 11; Fat: 0.09; Carb: 2.69; Protein: 0.24

Fresh Pineapple Salsa

Prep Time: 15 Minutes   Cook Time: 1 Hour   Serves: 6

Ingredients:

- 1 cup finely chopped fresh pineapple
- ¼ cup finely chopped red onion
- ¼ cup red bell pepper, chopped
- 1 jalapeño pepper, seeded and minced
- 1 tablespoon finely chopped fresh cilantro
- 1 tablespoon lime juice
- 1 clove garlic, minced (Optional)
- ½ teaspoon white sugar

- ½ teaspoon salt

Directions:

1. Mix pineapple, red onion, bell pepper, jalapeño, cilantro, lime juice, garlic, sugar, and salt together in a bowl until combined.
2. Cover with plastic wrap and refrigerate for 1 hour so flavors can meld.

Nutritional Value (Amount per Serving):

Calories: 33; Fat: 0.11; Carb: 8.27; Protein: 0.47

Easy-to-Make Apple Sandwich

Prep Time: 5 Minutes   Cook Time: 5 Minutes   Serves: 1

Ingredients:

- 1 ½ tablespoons creamy peanut butter (Optional)
- 2 slices apple
- 2 tablespoons granola, or more to taste

Directions:

1. Spread peanut butter over one side of one apple slice; top with granola. Place remaining apple slice atop the granola to finish the sandwich.
2. Cover and refrigerate until ready to eat.

Nutritional Value (Amount per Serving):

Calories: 580; Fat: 24.12; Carb: 89.02; Protein: 9.49

Ground Cherry Salsa

Prep Time: 30 Minutes   Cook Time: 5 Minutes   Serves: 4

Ingredients:

- 1 ½ limes, juiced, or more to taste
- 2 tablespoons finely chopped red onion
- ½ cup ground cherries, husked and halved
- ½ cup cherry tomatoes, quartered
- 1 jalapeno pepper, seeded and minced
- ½ finely chopped seeded cucumber
- 2 tablespoons finely chopped cilantro, or more to taste
- 1 dash passion fruit-jalapeno fruit vinegar (optional)
- salt to taste

Directions:

1. Mix lime juice and red onion together in a bowl and let stand for about 5

minutes, as this mellows the raw onion taste.

2. Add ground cherries, cherry tomatoes, jalapeno pepper, cucumber, cilantro, vinegar, and salt to the bowl and mix well.
3. Serve right away or cover and refrigerate until serving.

Nutritional Value (Amount per Serving):

Calories: 186; Fat: 12.58; Carb: 4.01; Protein: 14.03

Gorgonzola-Walnut Stuffed Dates

Prep Time: 15 Minutes   Cook Time: 15 Minutes   Serves: 36

Ingredients:

- 1 (3 ounce) package cream cheese, softened
- 3 ounces crumbled Gorgonzola cheese
- 36 pitted dates
- 36 walnut pieces

Directions:

1. Mix cream cheese and Gorgonzola cheese together in a bowl.
2. Cut a slit into each date so they can be spread flat. Spread cheese mixture into each date; top with a walnut piece.
3. Cover and refrigerate until ready to eat.

Nutritional Value (Amount per Serving):

Calories: 820; Fat: 79.64; Carb: 21.92; Protein: 19.12

Simple Roasted Chickpea Snack

Prep Time: 10 Minutes   Cook Time: 45 Minutes   Serves: 4

Ingredients:

- 2 tablespoons olive oil
- 1 tablespoon ground cumin
- 1 teaspoon garlic powder
- ½ teaspoon chili powder
- 1 pinch sea salt
- 1 pinch ground black pepper
- 1 dash crushed red pepper
- 1 (15 ounce) can chickpeas, rinsed and drained

Directions:

1. Preheat the oven to 350 degrees F.
2. Whisk oil, cumin, garlic powder, chili powder, sea salt, black pepper, and red pepper together in a small bowl; add chickpeas and toss to coat. Spread in a single layer on a baking sheet.
3. Roast in the preheated oven, stirring occasionally, until nicely browned

and slightly crispy, about 45 minutes.

Nutritional Value (Amount per Serving):

Calories: 166; Fat: 8.94; Carb: 17.78; Protein: 5.35

No-Bake Energy Bites

Prep Time: 15 Minutes   Cook Time: 1 Hour   Serves: 24

Ingredients:

- 1 cup rolled oats
- ½ cup miniature semisweet chocolate chips
- ½ cup ground flax seed
- ½ cup crunchy peanut butter
- ⅓ cup honey
- 1 teaspoon vanilla extract

Directions:

1. Blend milk, yogurt, banana, peanut butter, spinach, and ice cubes until smooth.
2. Stir oats, chocolate chips, flax seed, peanut butter, honey, and vanilla extract together in a bowl.
3. Roll dough into 24 balls with your hands. Arrange balls on a baking sheet and freeze until set, about 1 hour.

Nutritional Value (Amount per Serving):

Calories: 101; Fat: 5.8; Carb: 12.21; Protein: 3.29

Banana Oatmeal Protein Bars

Prep Time: 10 Minutes   Cook Time: 40 Minutes   Serves: 25

Ingredients:

- 2 cups gluten-free rolled oats
- 1 cup mashed banana
- ⅔ cup vanilla protein powder (such as Muscletech Whey Protein Plus)
- ½ cup peanut butter, slightly melted
- ½ cup sweetened dried cranberries (such as Craisins)
- ½ cup unsweetened flaked coconut (Optional)
- ½ cup chopped raw almonds
- ¼ cup brewed sweet and spicy black tea (such as Good Earth Sweet&Spicy
- 2 tablespoons chia seeds
- 1 ½ teaspoons ground cinnamon

- 1 teaspoon vanilla extract
- ¼ cup coconut, or to taste (Optional)

Directions:

1. Preheat oven to 350 degrees F. Grease an 8-inch square pan.
2. Mix oats, banana, protein powder, peanut butter, cranberries, 1/2 cup coconut, almonds, tea, chia seeds, cinnamon, and vanilla together in a large mixing bowl; spread into prepared pan. Top with 1/4 cup coconut.
3. Bake bars until lightly browned, 25 to 30 minutes. Set aside to cool until they set completely, at least 15 minutes.

Nutritional Value (Amount per Serving):

Calories: 68; Fat: 2.3; Carb: 12.9; Protein: 2.32

Carrot Chips

Prep Time: 10 Minutes   Cook Time: 12 Minutes   Serves: 4

Ingredients:

- 4 carrots, washed
- 2 teaspoons extra-virgin olive oil
- ¼ teaspoon salt

Directions:

1. Preheat oven to 350 degrees F. Put one rack on the highest level in the oven and another on the bottom.
2. Peel carrots into thin strips using a vegetable peeler; put into a large bowl. Drizzle olive oil over the carrot strips and toss to coat. Season with salt; toss again. Spread carrots onto 2 baking sheets in a single layer, preventing overlap.
3. Put one baking sheet on the top rack and the other on the bottom. Bake carrots in preheated oven for 6 minutes, switch racks, and continue baking until the carrots are crisp, about 6 minutes more. Cool chips until cool enough to handle before serving.

Nutritional Value (Amount per Serving):

Calories: 34; Fat: 1.12; Carb: 5.84; Protein: 0.58

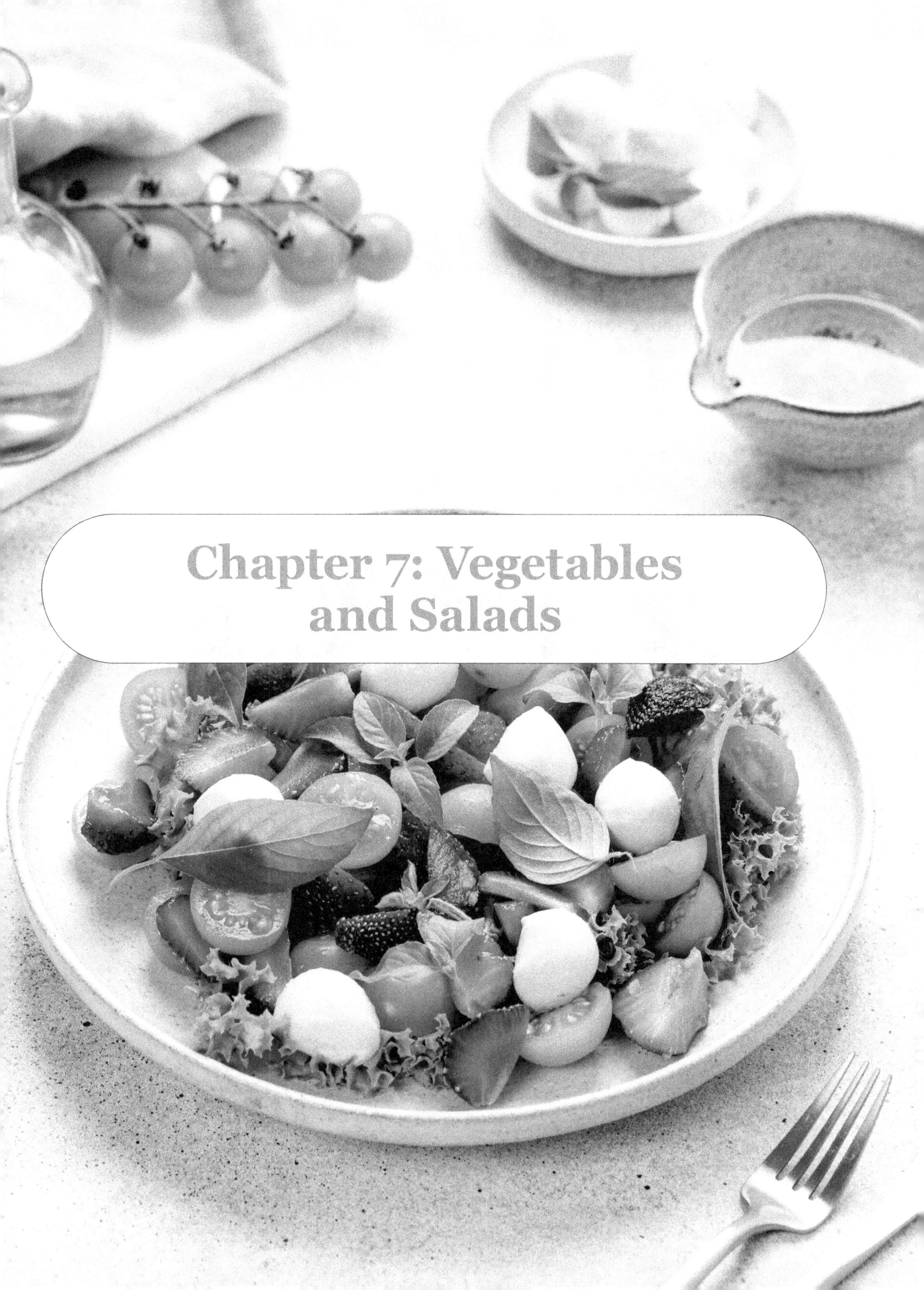

Chapter 7: Vegetables and Salads

Raw Cauliflower Salad

Prep Time: 20 Minutes   Cook Time: 2 Hours   Serves: 5

Ingredients:

- 4 cups cauliflower, thinly sliced
- 1 cup coarsely chopped olives
- ⅔ cup coarsely chopped green bell pepper (Optional)
- ½ cup chopped pimento peppers (Optional)
- ½ cup onion, chopped (Optional)
- 1 bunch celery stalks, thinly sliced
- ½ cup canola oil
- 3 tablespoons lemon juice
- 3 tablespoons red or white wine vinegar
- ½ teaspoon salt
- ¼ teaspoon white sugar
- ¼ teaspoon ground black pepper

Directions:

1. Combine cauliflower, olives, bell pepper, pimento peppers, onion, and celery in a large bowl.
2. Combine oil, lemon juice, vinegar, salt, sugar, and black pepper in a small jar with a lid. Close jar and shake until dressing is combined. Pour over vegetables.
3. Marinate cauliflower salad in the refrigerator for 2 to 4 hours.

Nutritional Value (Amount per Serving):

Calories: 271; Fat: 26.08; Carb: 8.9; Protein: 2.95

Orzo Salad

Prep Time: 30 Minutes   Cook Time: 8 Minutes   Serves: 6

Ingredients:

- 1½ cups dry orzo pasta
- 1 recipe Greek Salad Dressing
- 1 tablespoon red wine vinegar
- 1 tablespoon fresh lemon juice
- ½ teaspoon oregano
- ¼ teaspoon sea salt
- 2 Persian cucumbers, halved vertically, and sliced ¼-inch thick
- 2 cups halved cherry tomatoes
- 1 cup cooked chickpeas, drained, and rinsed

- 4 ounces feta cheese, cut into ¼-inch cubes
- ⅓ cup thinly sliced red onion
- ½ cup pitted Kalamata olives
- 1 cup fresh basil and/or mint leaves
- Freshly ground black pepper

1. Bring a large pot of salted water to a boil. Prepare the pasta according to the package directions, or until slightly past al dente. Drain the orzo and toss it with a little olive oil, so that it doesn't stick together. Spread onto a baking sheet to cool.
2. Prepare the Greek Salad Dressing and add in the red wine vinegar, lemon juice, oregano, and sea salt.
3. In a large bowl, toss together the cooked orzo, cucumbers, tomatoes, chickpeas, feta, red onion, and olives. Drizzle the dressing over the salad, add half the herbs, season with freshly ground black pepper, and toss to coat. Garnish with the remaining herbs and store in the fridge.

Nutritional Value (Amount per Serving):

Calories: 235; Fat: 9.38; Carb: 30.58; Protein: 8.2

Italian Romanesco Cauliflower Salad

Prep Time: 30 Minutes   Cook Time: 15 Minutes   Serves: 8

Ingredients:

- 2 pounds broccoli, broken into florets
- 1 head cauliflower, broken into florets
- 1 head Romanesco cauliflower, broken into florets
- 2 lemons, juiced
- 6 ½ tablespoons extra-virgin olive oil
- 1 clove garlic, minced
- 1 teaspoon chopped fresh oregano
- salt and ground black pepper to taste
- 10 green Italian olives, or more to taste
- 10 black Italian olives, or more to taste
- 2 papaccelle (pickled sweet peppers), cut into strips

Directions:

1. Bring a large pot of lightly salted water to a boil. Add broccoli and cook uncovered until just tender, about 1 1/2 minutes. Remove to a plate with a slotted spoon, reserving water, and let cool.
2. Stir cauliflower into the boiling water. Cook until just tender, about 3 minutes. Remove to a plate with a slotted spoon, reserving water, and let

cool.

3. Stir Romanesco cauliflower into the boiling water. Cook until just tender, about 3 minutes. Drain and let cool.
4. Whisk lemon juice, olive oil, garlic, oregano, salt, and pepper together in a small bowl to make dressing.
5. Layer broccoli, cauliflower, and Romanesco cauliflower in round serving containers. Decorate each layer with green and black olives and strips of papaccelle. Pour dressing on top, and store in the fridge.

Nutritional Value (Amount per Serving):

Calories: 103; Fat: 6.47; Carb: 9.21; Protein: 5.45

Mediterranean Quinoa Salad

Prep Time: 20 Minutes   Cook Time: 2 Hours   Serves: 6

Ingredients:

- 3 cups cooked quinoa
- 1 recipe Roasted Tomatoes
- 2 cups arugula
- 1 cup sliced Persian cucumbers
- 1 cup mixed basil & mint
- ¾ cup Kalamata olives, pitted and sliced
- ½ cup diced red onion
- ⅓ cup toasted pine nuts
- 1 recipe Italian Dressing, plus 2 additional garlic cloves, grated
- ½ teaspoon sea salt
- Freshly ground black pepper
- Pinches of red pepper flakes
- 1 cup roasted chickpeas

Directions:

1. In a large bowl, combine the quinoa, roasted tomatoes, arugula, cucumbers, herbs, olives, onion, and pine nuts.
2. Toss to combine, then drizzle with the dressing and toss again. Sprinkle with salt, pepper, and a few pinches of red pepper flakes, and toss again. Top with the roasted chickpeas and store in the fridge.

Note: the quinoa and roasted tomatoes can be made up to 3 days in advance, and stored in the fridge until ready to use.

Nutritional Value (Amount per Serving):

Calories: 329; Fat: 13.38; Carb: 44.94; Protein: 10.42

Greek Salad

Prep Time: 10 Minutes   Cook Time: 20 Minutes   Serves:6

Ingredients:

- 1 head romaine lettuce- rinsed, dried and chopped
- 1 cucumber, sliced
- 2 large tomatoes, chopped
- 1 (6 ounce) can pitted black olives
- 1 green bell pepper, chopped
- 1 red bell pepper, chopped
- 1 red onion, thinly sliced
- 1 cup crumbled feta cheese
- 6 tablespoons olive oil
- 1 lemon, juiced
- 1 teaspoon dried oregano
- ground black pepper to taste

Directions:

1. Combine romaine, cucumber, tomatoes, olives, bell peppers, and red onion in a large bowl; sprinkle with feta cheese.
2. Whisk olive oil, lemon juice, oregano, and black pepper together in a small bowl. Pour dressing over salad, toss well to combine, and store in the fridge.

Nutritional Value (Amount per Serving):

Calories: 277; Fat: 23.75; Carb: 9.98; Protein: 8.47

Spinach Pomegranate Salad

Prep Time: 10 Minutes   Cook Time: 10 Minutes   Serves:4

Ingredients:

- 1 (10 ounce) bag baby spinach leaves, rinsed and drained
- ½ cup walnut pieces
- ½ cup crumbled feta
- ¼ medium red onion, sliced very thin
- ¼ cup alfalfa sprouts (Optional)
- ½ cup pomegranate seeds, or to taste
- 4 tablespoons balsamic vinaigrette

Directions:

1. Gather all ingredients.
2. Place spinach into a salad bowl. Top with walnuts, feta, red onion, alfalfa

sprouts, and pomegranate seeds.

3. Drizzle with vinaigrette and store in the fridge.

Calories: 182; Fat: 11.33; Carb: 16.07; Protein: 8.21

Classic Caesar Salad

Prep Time: 20 Minutes   Cook Time: 20 Minutes   Serves:2

Ingredients:

- 3 anchovy fillets
- 2 cloves garlic, finely chopped
- ½ lemon, juiced
- 2 tablespoons red wine vinegar
- 1 large egg yolk
- 1 tablespoon Dijon mustard
- 1 dash Worcestershire sauce
- ¼ cup olive oil
- salt and ground black pepper to taste
- ½ head romaine lettuce, chopped
- ¼ cup grated Parmesan cheese
- 2 tablespoons croutons

Directions:

1. Gather all ingredients.
2. To make the dressing: Mash anchovy fillets and garlic in a large salad bowl. Add lemon juice, red wine vinegar, Dijon mustard, egg yolk, and Worcestershire sauce; whisk until smooth and creamy. Gradually stream in olive oil while whisking constantly. Season with salt and black pepper.
3. Make salad: Gently mix romaine lettuce and Parmesan cheese into dressing until thoroughly coated.
4. Serve salad topped with croutons.
5. Store the salad and the dressing separately in the fridge if not eating right away.

Nutritional Value (Amount per Serving):

Calories: 392; Fat: 34.07; Carb: 14.09; Protein: 9.68

Simple Cranberry Spinach Salad

Prep Time: 5 Minutes   Cook Time: 5 Minutes   Serves:4

Ingredients:

- 1 (6 ounce) package fresh spinach
- ⅓ cup dried cranberries
- ⅓ cup chopped walnuts
- ⅓ cup raspberry walnut vinaigrette
- 1 tablespoon finely shredded Romano cheese

Directions:

1. Combine the spinach, cranberries, walnuts, vinaigrette, and Romano cheese in a large bowl; toss until spinach is evenly coated.
2. To store in the fridge: keep the vinaigrette separately from the rest of the salad ingredients. Mix before eating.

Nutritional Value (Amount per Serving):

Calories: 95; Fat: 4.97; Carb: 11.41; Protein: 3.57

Butter Lettuce Salad with Dijon-Tarragon Vinaigrette

Prep Time: 15 Minutes   Cook Time: 15 Minutes   Serves:6

Ingredients:

- 3 tablespoons extra-virgin olive oil
- 2 tablespoons white wine vinegar
- 2 tablespoons minced shallot
- 1/2 tablespoon Dijon mustard
- 1/2 tablespoon chopped fresh tarragon
- 1/2 teaspoon salt
- 1/2 teaspoon black pepper
- 1 (5- to 6-oz.) package butter lettuce, torn or chopped
- 1 cup sugar snap peas, halved on the bias
- 4 radishes, thinly sliced

Directions:

1. For vinaigrette, shake together oil, vinegar, shallot, mustard, tarragon, salt, and pepper in a Mason jar until emulsified, about 30 seconds.
2. Put lettuce, peas, and radishes in a serving bowl. Add vinaigrette; toss to coat.
3. Store in fridge.

Nutritional Value (Amount per Serving):

Calories: 269; Fat: 24.44; Carb: 11.9; Protein: 2.46

Stone Fruit and Tomato Salad

Prep Time: 10 Minutes   Cook Time: 5 Minutes   Serves: 4

Ingredients:

- 1 fresh peach, chopped
- 2 plums, pitted and chopped
- 1 cup chopped tomato
- 1 cup pitted and halved cherries
- 2 tablespoons chopped fresh parsley
- 1 teaspoon lemon zest
- 1 tablespoon lemon juice
- 1 clove garlic, minced
- ¼ teaspoon salt
- ⅛ teaspoon ground black pepper
- 1 tablespoon extra-virgin olive oil

Directions:

1. Stir together peach, plums, tomato, cherries, parsley, lemon zest, lemon juice, minced garlic, salt, and black pepper in a large bowl until combined. Let stand at least 5 minutes to allow flavors to blend. Drizzle with olive oil and stir to combine.
2. Store in the fridge.

Nutritional Value (Amount per Serving):

Calories: 85; Fat: 1.72; Carb: 18.09; Protein: 1.16

Green Salad

Prep Time: 15 Minutes   Cook Time: 15 Minutes   Serves:8

Ingredients:

- ½ cup chopped onion
- ½ cup chopped green bell pepper
- 2 (10 ounce) packages mixed salad greens
- 4 thinly sliced chicken deli meat, chopped
- 1 tomato, chopped
- ¼ teaspoon onion powder
- 3 dashes garlic powder
- 2 pinches salt and ground black pepper to taste
- 3 tablespoons balsamic vinaigrette salad dressing

Directions:

1. Place onion and bell pepper in a microwave-safe bowl; heat in microwave on high until soft, about 1 to 2 minutes. Set aside to cool.
2. Combine onion, bell pepper, salad greens, deli meat, and tomato in a large salad bowl. Sprinkle with onion powder, garlic powder, salt, and black pepper; toss well to mix.
3. Pour on salad dressing; toss well and serve.

Calories: 477; Fat: 21.98; Carb: 4.68; Protein: 61.66

Arugula Beet Salad

Prep Time: 10 Minutes   Cook Time: 40 Minutes   Serves:4

Ingredients:

- 3 large beets, peeled and cut into cubes
- 2 tablespoons olive oil, divided
- ½ teaspoon coarse salt, divided
- ¼ teaspoon ground black pepper, divided
- 1 bunch arugula, torn
- ⅓ cup walnuts or pecans
- ¼ cup balsamic vinegar

Directions:

1. Preheat the oven to 425 degrees F.
2. Mix beets, 1 tablespoon olive oil, 1/4 teaspoon salt, and 1/8 teaspoon black pepper together on a baking sheet.
3. Roast in the preheated oven until beets are tender, about 40 minutes.
4. Mix roasted beets, arugula, walnuts, balsamic vinegar, 1 tablespoon olive oil, 1/4 teaspoon salt, and 1/8 teaspoon pepper together in a bowl until well combined.

Nutritional Value (Amount per Serving):

Calories: 151; Fat: 11.33; Carb: 10.68; Protein: 2.77

Jamie's Cranberry Spinach Salad

Prep Time: 10 Minutes   Cook Time: 5 Minutes   Serves:8

Ingredients:

- 1 tablespoon butter
- ¾ cup almonds, blanched and slivered
- 1 pound spinach, rinsed and torn into bite-size pieces
- 1 cup dried cranberries
- ½ cup vegetable oil
- ½ cup white sugar
- ¼ cup cider vinegar
- ¼ cup white wine vinegar
- 2 tablespoons toasted sesame seeds

- 1 tablespoon poppy seeds
- 2 teaspoons minced onion
- ¼ teaspoon paprika

1. Melt butter in a medium saucepan over medium heat. Cook and stir almonds in butter until lightly toasted. Remove from heat and let cool.
2. Make dressing: Whisk together oil, sugar, cider vinegar, white wine vinegar, sesame seeds, poppy seeds, minced onion, and paprika in a medium bowl.
3. Combine spinach with toasted almonds and cranberries in a large serving bowl. Pour dressing over spinach mixture; toss well.

Nutritional Value (Amount per Serving):

Calories: 236; Fat: 19.27; Carb: 15.19; Protein: 3.23

BLT Salad

Prep Time: 15 Minutes   Cook Time: 10 Minutes   Serves:6

Ingredients:

- 1 pound bacon
- ¾ cup mayonnaise
- ¼ cup milk
- 1 teaspoon garlic powder
- ⅛ teaspoon ground black pepper
- salt to taste
- 1 head romaine lettuce - rinsed, dried and shredded
- 2 large tomatoes, chopped
- 2 cups seasoned croutons

Directions:

1. Place bacon in a large skillet and cook over medium-high heat, turning occasionally, until evenly browned, about 10 minutes. Drain bacon slices on paper towels; crumble and set aside.
2. Combine mayonnaise, milk, garlic powder, and black pepper together in a blender or food processor; blend until smooth. Season with salt.
3. Combine lettuce, crumbled bacon, tomatoes, and croutons in a large salad bowl. Toss with dressing, and serve immediately.

Nutritional Value (Amount per Serving):

Calories: 409; Fat: 33.15; Carb: 20.1; Protein: 13.14

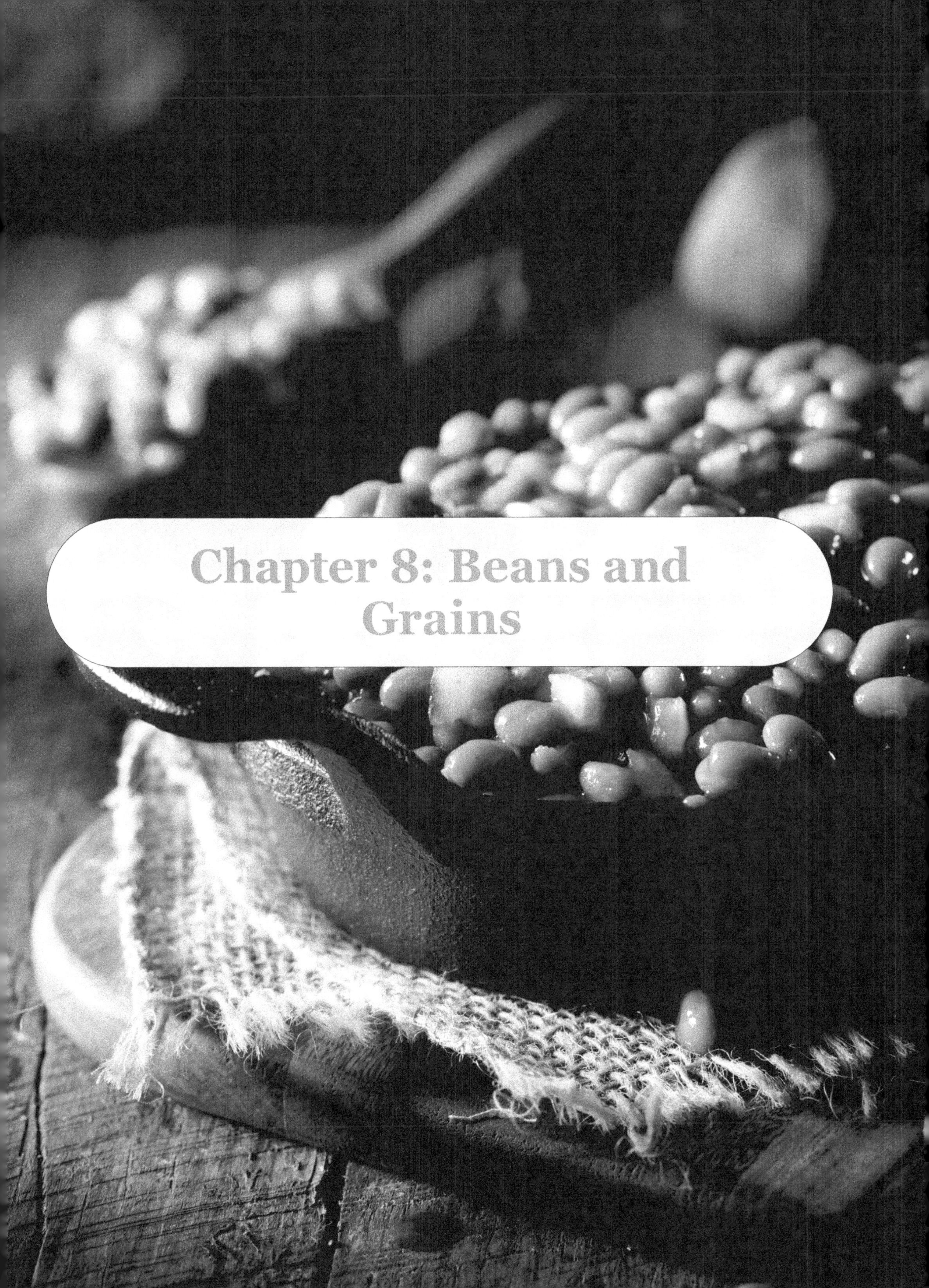

Chapter 8: Beans and Grains

Prep Time: 10 Minutes   Cook Time: 10 Minutes   Serves: 1

Ingredients:

- ¾ cup canned black beans, rinsed
- ⅔ cup cooked quinoa
- ¼ cup hummus
- 1 tablespoon lime juice
- ¼ medium avocado, diced
- 3 tablespoons pico de gallo
- 2 tablespoons chopped fresh cilantro

Directions:

1. Combine beans and quinoa in a bowl. Stir hummus and lime juice together in a small bowl; thin with water to desired consistency. Drizzle the hummus dressing over the beans and quinoa. Top with avocado, pico de gallo and cilantro.
2. Assemble Buddha bowl up to 1 day in advance, with dressing on the side. To prevent avocado from browning if making ahead, toss with a squeeze of lime juice after dicing.

Nutritional Value (Amount per Serving):

Calories: 853; Fat: 17.12; Carb: 139.66; Protein: 40.98

Chicken & White Bean Soup

Prep Time: 25 Minutes   Cook Time: 25 Minutes   Serves: 6

Ingredients:

- 2 teaspoons extra-virgin olive oil
- 2 leeks, white and light green parts only, cut into 1/4-inch rounds
- 1 tablespoon chopped fresh sage, or 1/4 teaspoon dried
- 2 14-ounce cans reduced-sodium chicken broth
- 2 cups water
- 1 15-ounce can cannellini beans, rinsed
- 1 2-pound roasted chicken, skin discarded, meat removed from bones and shredded (4 cups)

Directions:

1. Heat oil in a Dutch oven over medium-high heat. Add leeks and cook, stirring often, until soft, about 3 minutes. Stir in sage and continue cooking until aromatic, about 30 seconds. Stir in broth and water, increase heat to high, cover and bring to a boil. Add beans and chicken and cook,

uncovered, stirring occasionally, until heated through, about 3 minutes.

2. Cover and refrigerate for up to 2 days.

Nutritional Value (Amount per Serving):

Calories: 415; Fat: 21.93; Carb: 9.01; Protein: 44.39

Provencal White Beans

Prep Time: 10 Minutes   Cook Time: 40 Minutes   Serves: 8

Ingredients:

- 4 (15 ounce) cans great northern white beans
- 1 quart chicken stock
- 1/4 cup olive oil
- 2 cups chopped yellow onions
- 1 cup medium-diced carrots
- 1 cup medium-diced celery
- 1/4 cup chopped fresh parsley, plus extra for garnish
- 2 tablespoons minced fresh rosemary
- 2 tablespoons minced fresh thyme
- 1 tablespoon minced garlic
- 1/3 cup freshly grated Parmesan cheese

Directions:

1. Pour beans with their liquid and chicken stock into a large saucepan, and bring to a boil. Reduce the heat and simmer until tender but not mushy, about 15 minutes. Drain, reserving the stock.
2. Heat olive oil in a large skillet over low heat. Add onions, diced carrots, and celery, and cook until tender, 10 to 15 minutes. Stir in parsley, rosemary, thyme, and garlic, and cook until fragrant, about 1 minute.
3. Add beans and 2 cups of reserved cooking stock to the skillet. If you don't have enough liquid, add additional stock or water to make 2 cups.
4. Simmer until the stock is reduced and makes a little sauce, about 15 minutes. Add more stock if necessary.
5. Sprinkle with Parmesan cheese and garnish with chopped parsley to serve.
6. Cover and refrigerate for up to 2 days.

Nutritional Value (Amount per Serving):

Calories: 422; Fat: 13.18; Carb: 38; Protein: 37.72

Rice & Bean Freezer Burritos

Prep Time: 35 Minutes   Cook Time: 35 Minutes   Serves: 8

- 2 (15 ounce) cans low-sodium black or pinto beans, rinsed
- 4 teaspoons chili powder
- 1 teaspoon ground cumin
- 2 cups shredded sharp Cheddar cheese
- 1 cup chopped grape tomatoes
- 4 scallions, chopped
- ¼ cup chopped pickled jalapeños
- 2 tablespoons chopped fresh cilantro
- 8 8-inch whole-wheat tortillas, at room temperature
- 2 cups cooked brown rice

1. Mash beans in a large bowl with chili powder and cumin until almost smooth. Add cheese, tomatoes, scallions, jalapeños and cilantro; stir to combine.
2. Spread about 1/2 cup of the filling on the bottom third of each tortilla and top with about 1/4 cup rice. Roll up snugly, tucking in the ends as you go. If serving immediately, transfer to a microwave-safe plate, cover with a paper towel and microwave on High until steaming hot, 1 to 2 minutes. If freezing, wrap each burrito in foil. Freeze for up to 3 months.
3. To heat: Remove a burrito from the foil and place on a microwave-safe plate. Cover with a paper towel and microwave on High until steaming hot, 1 1/2 to 2 1/2 minutes.

Calories: 1274; Fat: 37.84; Carb: 194.25; Protein: 40.87

Best Black Beans

Prep Time: 5 Minutes   Cook Time: 10 Minutes   Serves: 4

- 1 (16 ounce) can black beans, undrained
- 1 small onion, chopped
- 1 clove garlic, chopped
- 1 tablespoon chopped fresh cilantro
- ¼ teaspoon cayenne pepper
- salt to taste

1. Gather all ingredients.
2. Combine beans, onion, and garlic in a medium saucepan; bring to a boil.
3. Reduce heat to medium-low. Stir in cilantro, cayenne, and salt. Simmer for 5 minutes.
4. Remove from pot, sprinkle with cilantro, and serve or store in refrigerator.

Calories: 395; Fat: 1.65; Carb: 72.68; Protein: 24.75

Edamame & Veggie Rice Bowl

Prep Time: 5 Minutes   Cook Time: 5 Minutes   Serves: 1

Ingredients:

- ½ cup cooked brown rice (see associated recipes)
- 1 cup roasted vegetables (see associated recipes)
- ¼ cup edamame
- ¼ avocado, diced
- 2 tablespoons sliced scallions
- 2 tablespoons chopped fresh cilantro
- 2 tablespoons Citrus-Lime Vinaigrette (see associated recipes)

Directions:

1. Arrange rice, veggies, edamame and avocado in a 4-cup sealable container or bowl. Top with scallions and cilantro. Drizzle with vinaigrette just before serving.
2. Refrigerate dressing and bowl separately for up to 5 days.

Nutritional Value (Amount per Serving):

Calories: 2290; Fat: 229.41; Carb: 68.7; Protein: 11.36

Rainbow Grain Bowl with Cashew Sauce

Prep Time: 20 Minutes   Cook Time: 20 Minutes   Serves: 1

Ingredients:

- ¾ cup unsalted cashews
- ½ cup water
- ¼ cup packed parsley leaves
- 1 tablespoon lemon juice or cider vinegar
- 1 tablespoon extra-virgin olive oil
- ½ teaspoon reduced-sodium tamari or soy sauce (see Tip)
- ¼ teaspoon salt
- ½ cup cooked lentils
- ½ cup cooked quinoa
- ½ cup shredded red cabbage
- ¼ cup grated raw beet
- ¼ cup chopped bell pepper

- ¼ cup grated carrot
- ¼ cup sliced cucumber
- 1 tablespoon Toasted chopped cashews for garnish

Directions:

1. Blend cashews, water, parsley, lemon juice (or vinegar), oil, tamari (or soy sauce) and salt in a blender until smooth.
2. Place lentils and quinoa in the center of a shallow serving bowl. Top with cabbage, beet, pepper, carrot and cucumber. Spoon 2 tablespoons of the cashew sauce over the top (save extra sauce for another use). Garnish with cashews, if desired.
3. Refrigerate for up to 2 days.

Nutritional Value (Amount per Serving):

Calories: 1582; Fat: 111.87; Carb: 115.85; Protein: 51.11

Instant Pot Black Beans

Prep Time: 5 Minutes   Cook Time: 45 Minutes   Serves:7

Ingredients:

- 1 ¼ cups dry black beans

Directions:

1. Pour beans into a multi-functional pressure cooker. Cover with a few inches of cool water. Close and lock the lid. Select Manual; set timer for 21 minutes on high pressure according to manufacturer's instructions. Allow 10 to 15 minutes for pressure to build.
2. Release pressure using the natural-release method according to manufacturer's instructions, 10 to 40 minutes. Unlock and remove the lid. Drain beans and let cool.
3. Refrigerate for up to 3 days.

Nutritional Value (Amount per Serving):

Calories: 40; Fat: 0.11; Carb: 7.44; Protein: 2.5

Muesli

Prep Time: 10 Minutes   Cook Time: 10 Minutes   Serves:16

Ingredients:

- 4 ½ cups rolled oats
- 1 cup raisins
- ½ cup toasted wheat germ
- ½ cup wheat bran
- ½ cup oat bran
- ½ cup chopped walnuts

- ¼ cup packed brown sugar
- ¼ cup raw sunflower seeds

Directions:

1. Combine oats, raisins, wheat germ, wheat bran, oat bran, walnuts, brown sugar, and sunflower seeds in a large bowl; mix well.
2. Store muesli in an airtight container at room temperature for up to 2 months.

Nutritional Value (Amount per Serving):

Calories: 131; Fat: 5.25; Carb: 26.66; Protein: 7.04

Quinoa and Black Beans

Prep Time: 15 Minutes   Cook Time: 35 Minutes   Serves: 10

Ingredients:

- 1 teaspoon vegetable oil
- 1 onion, chopped
- 3 cloves garlic, chopped
- ¾ cup quinoa
- 1 ½ cups vegetable broth
- 1 teaspoon ground cumin
- ¼ teaspoon cayenne pepper
- salt and ground black pepper to taste
- 1 cup frozen corn kernels
- 2 (15 ounce) cans black beans, rinsed and drained
- ½ cup chopped fresh cilantro

Directions:

1. Gather all ingredients.
2. Heat oil in a large saucepan over medium heat. Add onion and garlic; cook and stir until lightly browned, about 10 minutes.
3. Mix quinoa into onion mixture and cover with vegetable broth; season with cumin, cayenne pepper, salt, and pepper.
4. Bring to a boil; cover, reduce heat, and simmer until quinoa is tender and broth is absorbed, about 20 minutes.
5. Stir in frozen corn and continue to simmer until heated through, about 5 minutes. Mix in black beans and cilantro.
6. Store in freezer for up to 2 months.

Nutritional Value (Amount per Serving):

Calories: 225; Fat: 2.11; Carb: 40.7; Protein: 11.83

Boston Baked Beans

Prep Time: 10 Minutes   Cook Time: 4 Hours 10 Minutes   Serves: 6

Ingredients:

- 2 cups dry navy beans, soaked overnight
- ½ pound uncooked bacon strips
- 1 medium onion, diced
- ½ cup ketchup
- 3 tablespoons molasses
- ¼ cup brown sugar
- 1 tablespoon Worcestershire sauce
- 2 teaspoons salt
- ¼ teaspoon ground black pepper
- ¼ teaspoon dry mustard

Directions:

1. Transfer soaked navy beans and soaking water to a saucepan.
2. Bring to a boil. Reduce heat and simmer until nearly tender, approximately 1 to 2 hours. Drain and reserve the cooking liquid.
3. Preheat the oven to 325 degrees F.
4. Arrange 1/2 of the beans in the bottom of a 2-quart casserole dish. Place 1/2 of the bacon strips over the beans and sprinkle 1/2 of the onions over top. Repeat layers once more.
5. Combine ketchup, molasses, brown sugar, Worcestershire sauce, salt, pepper, and dry mustard in a large saucepan over medium heat; bring to a boil.
6. Pour sauce over the beans. Pour in just enough reserved cooking liquid to cover the beans. Cover the casserole dish with a lid or aluminum foil.
7. Bake in the preheated oven for 1 1/2 hours. Remove the lid and continue to cook, checking every 1/2 hour or so and adding more cooking liquid if necessary to prevent the beans from getting too dry, until beans are soft and tender, 1 1/2 to 2 1/2 more hours.
8. Serve hot and enjoy!

Nutritional Value (Amount per Serving):

Calories: 223; Fat: 11.45; Carb: 28.99; Protein: 5.07

Baked Grains Pilaf

Prep Time: 15 Minutes   Cook Time: 40 Minutes   Serves: 8

Ingredients:

- 1 tablespoon vegetable oil
- 1 onion, chopped

- 3 stalks celery, chopped
- ½ cup chopped bell pepper
- ½ cup corn kernels
- ¾ cup millet
- ¾ cup quinoa
- 1 teaspoon salt
- 3 cups low-sodium chicken stock

Directions:

1. Preheat oven to 350 degrees F.
2. Heat oil in a skillet over medium heat; cook and stir onion, celery, bell pepper, and corn in the hot oil until softened, about 10 minutes.
3. Mix onion mixture, millet, quinoa, and salt together in an 8x8-inch casserole dish; pour in chicken stock. Cover dish with aluminum foil.
4. Bake in the preheated oven until grains are tender and have absorbed all the liquid, about 30 minutes.

Nutritional Value (Amount per Serving):

Calories: 174; Fat: 4.17; Carb: 28.25; Protein: 6.61

Quick Black Beans and Rice

Prep Time: 5 Minutes   Cook Time: 20 Minutes   Serves: 4

Ingredients:

- 1 tablespoon vegetable oil
- 1 onion, chopped
- 1 (15 ounce) can black beans, undrained
- 1 (14.5 ounce) can stewed tomatoes
- 1 teaspoon dried oregano
- ½ teaspoon garlic powder
- 1 ½ cups uncooked instant brown rice

Directions:

1. Heat oil over medium-high in a large saucepan. Add onion; cook and stir until tender. Add beans, tomatoes, oregano, and garlic powder. Bring to a boil.
2. Stir in rice. Cover; reduce heat and simmer for 5 minutes. Remove from heat; let stand 5 minutes before serving.

Nutritional Value (Amount per Serving):

Calories: 558; Fat: 6.12; Carb: 101.55; Protein: 26.81

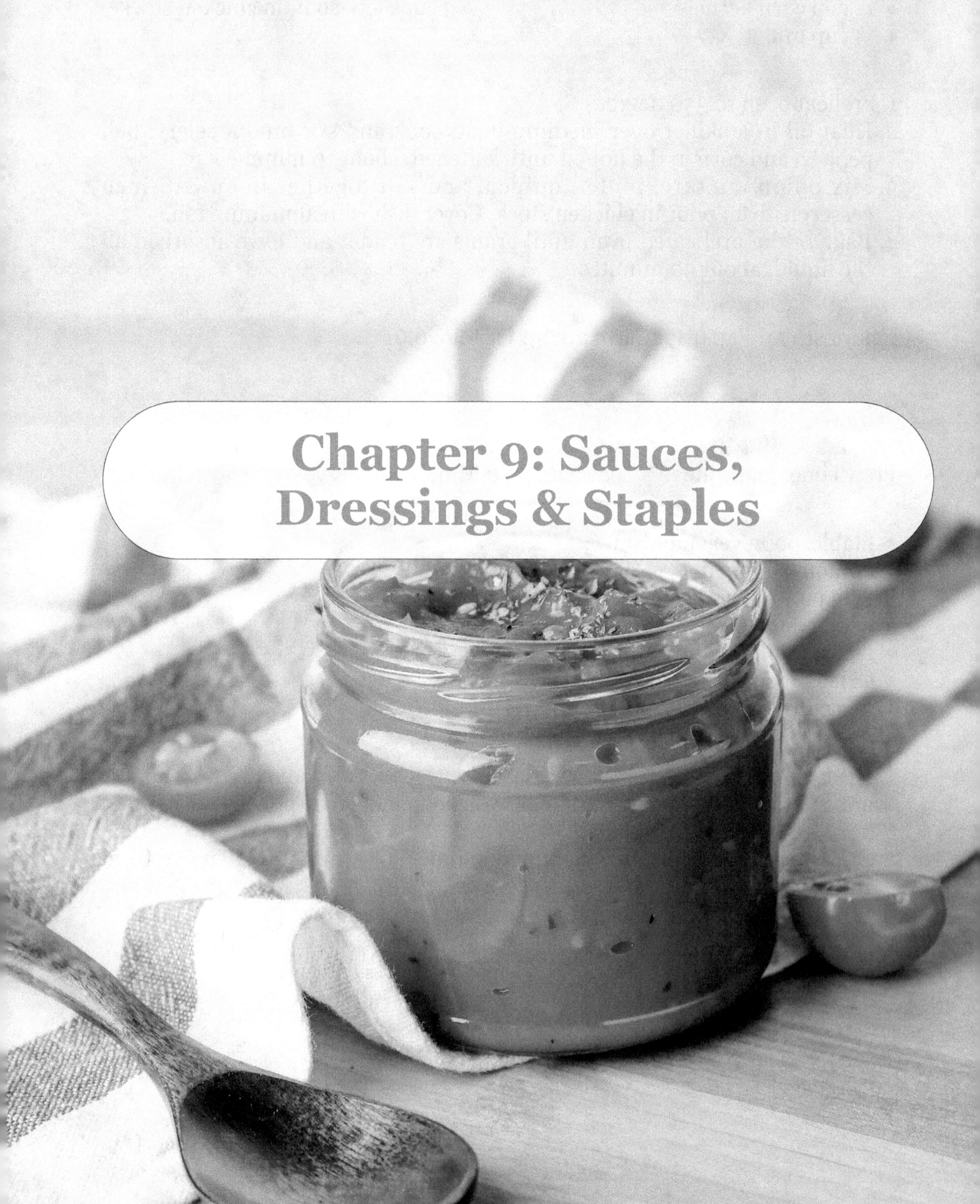

Chapter 9: Sauces, Dressings & Staples

White Sauce

Prep Time: 5 Minutes   Cook Time: 10 Minutes   Serves: 8

Ingredients:

- 2 tablespoons butter
- 2 tablespoons all-purpose flour
- 1 cup milk, or more as needed

Directions:

1. Melt butter in a small saucepan over medium-low heat. Whisk in flour to form a thick paste; cook and stir until golden in color, about 5 to 7 minutes.
2. Whisk in 1 cup milk; cook and stir until thickened, about 5 minutes. Add more milk to reach desired consistency. Store in an airtight container.

Nutritional Value (Amount per Serving):

Calories: 51; Fat: 3.9; Carb: 2.95; Protein: 1.19

Easy Coleslaw Dressing

Prep Time: 5 Minutes   Cook Time: 5 Minutes   Serves: 6

Ingredients:

- ½ cup mayonnaise
- 2 tablespoons white sugar
- 1 ½ tablespoons lemon juice
- 1 tablespoon vinegar
- ½ teaspoon ground black pepper
- ¼ teaspoon salt

Directions:

1. Gather all ingredients.
2. Whisk mayonnaise, sugar, lemon juice, vinegar, pepper, and salt together in a bowl until smooth and creamy.
3. Store in an airtight container.

Nutritional Value (Amount per Serving):

Calories: 70; Fat: 6.57; Carb: 1.38; Protein: 1.31

Absolutely Fabulous Greek Salad Dressing

Prep Time: 10 Minutes   Cook Time: 10 Minutes   Serves: 120

Ingredients:

- 1 ½ quarts olive oil
- ⅓ cup garlic powder
- ⅓ cup dried oregano
- ⅓ cup dried basil
- ¼ cup ground black pepper
- ¼ cup salt
- ¼ cup onion powder
- ¼ cup Dijon-style mustard

- 2 quarts red wine vinegar

1. Gather all ingredients.
2. Mix olive oil, garlic powder, oregano, basil, pepper, salt, onion powder, and Dijon-style mustard together in a very large container. Pour in vinegar slowly while mixing vigorously until well blended.
3. Pour over salad or store in an airtight container at room temperature.

Nutritional Value (Amount per Serving):

Calories: 4; Fat: 0.17; Carb: 0.65; Protein: 0.13

Homemade Ranch Dressing

Prep Time: 5 Minutes   Cook Time: 30 Minutes   Serves: 12

Ingredients:

- 1 cup mayonnaise
- ½ cup sour cream
- ½ teaspoon dried chives
- ½ teaspoon dried parsley
- ½ teaspoon dried dill weed
- ¼ teaspoon garlic powder
- ¼ teaspoon onion powder
- ⅛ teaspoon salt
- ⅛ teaspoon ground black pepper

Directions:

1. Gather all ingredients.
2. Whisk mayonnaise, sour cream, chives, parsley, dill, garlic powder, onion powder, salt, and pepper together in a large bowl until well-combined.
3. Store in an airtight container.

Nutritional Value (Amount per Serving):

Calories: 78; Fat: 7.38; Carb: 1.46; Protein: 1.56

Italian Dressing Mix

Prep Time: 5 Minutes   Cook Time: 5 Minutes   Serves: 16

Ingredients:

- 2 tablespoons dried oregano
- 2 tablespoons salt
- 1 tablespoon dried parsley
- 1 tablespoon garlic salt
- 1 tablespoon onion powder
- 1 tablespoon white sugar
- 1 teaspoon ground black pepper
- 1 teaspoon dried basil
- ¼ teaspoon dried thyme
- ¼ teaspoon celery salt

Directions:

1. Mix together oregano, salt, parsley, garlic salt, onion powder, sugar,

pepper, basil, thyme, and celery salt in a bowl.
2. Store in a tightly sealed container until ready to use.

Calories: 9; Fat: 0.13; Carb: 2.15; Protein: 0.33

Lebanese Lemon Salad Dressing

Prep Time: 20 Minutes   Cook Time: 20 Minutes   Serves: 6

Ingredients:

- ½ cup fresh lemon juice
- ½ cup mild extra-virgin olive oil
- 3 cloves garlic, minced
- 1 teaspoon kosher salt
- ground black pepper to taste

Directions:

1. In a medium bowl, whisk together the lemon juice, olive oil, garlic, salt and pepper.
2. Store in an airtight container. Stir just before serving.

Nutritional Value (Amount per Serving):

Calories: 80; Fat: 7.8; Carb: 2.61; Protein: 0.39

Honey Mustard Dressing

Prep Time: 5 Minutes   Cook Time: 5 Minutes   Serves: 3

Ingredients:

- ¼ cup mayonnaise
- 1 tablespoon prepared mustard
- 1 tablespoon honey
- ½ tablespoon lemon juice

Directions:

1. Gather all ingredients.
2. Whisk mayonnaise, mustard, honey, and lemon juice together in a small bowl.
3. Store covered in the refrigerator. Serve as a dip or salad dressing.

Nutritional Value (Amount per Serving):

Calories: 89; Fat: 6.54; Carb: 6.86; Protein: 1.41

Poppyseed Dressing

Prep Time: 15 Minutes   Cook Time: 15 Minutes   Serves: 14

Ingredients:

- ½ cup white vinegar
- ⅓ cup white sugar

- 1 teaspoon grated onion
- 1 teaspoon ground dry mustard
- 1 teaspoon salt
- 1 cup vegetable oil
- 1 tablespoon poppy seeds

Directions:

1. Place vinegar, sugar, onion, mustard, and salt into a blender or food processor; blend for 20 seconds. With the blender running, gradually add oil in a thin steady stream until combined.
2. Transfer dressing to a bowl and stir in poppy seeds.

Nutritional Value (Amount per Serving):

Calories: 158; Fat: 16.77; Carb: 2.66; Protein: 0.45

Cilantro Lime Salad Dressing

Prep Time: 10 Minutes   Cook Time: 10 Minutes   Serves: 16

Ingredients:

- 1 medium jalapeno pepper, seeded and coarsely chopped
- 1 clove garlic
- ¾ teaspoon minced fresh ginger root
- ⅓ cup honey
- ¼ cup lime juice
- ¼ cup packed cilantro leaves
- 2 teaspoons balsamic vinegar
- ½ teaspoon salt, or to taste
- ½ cup extra-virgin olive oil

Directions:

1. Pulse jalapeño, garlic, and ginger in a food processor until finely chopped. Add honey, lime juice, cilantro, vinegar, and salt; pulse 3 to 4 times to blend. Pour oil in slowly, with the processor running, until dressing is smooth.
2. Store in an airtight container. Taste and season with salt if needed before serving.

Nutritional Value (Amount per Serving):

Calories: 50; Fat: 2.91; Carb: 6.34; Protein: 0.09

Asian Ginger Dressing

Prep Time: 5 Minutes   Cook Time: 5 Minutes   Serves: 20

Ingredients:

- ¾ cup olive oil
- ½ cup soy sauce

- ⅓ cup rice vinegar
- ¼ cup water
- 3 tablespoons honey

- 3 cloves garlic, minced
- 2 tablespoons minced fresh ginger root

Directions:

1. Combine olive oil, soy sauce, rice vinegar, water, honey, garlic, and ginger in a 1-pint glass jar. Cover the jar with a tight-fitting lid; shake well.
2. Remove the lid, then heat the jar in the microwave until honey is dissolved, about 1 minute. Allow to cool.
3. Shake well before serving. Store covered in the refrigerator.

Nutritional Value (Amount per Serving):

Calories: 102; Fat: 9.26; Carb: 4.47; Protein: 0.5

Authentic Thousand Island Dressing

Prep Time: 20 Minutes   Cook Time: 5 Minutes   Serves: 16

Ingredients:

- 3 eggs
- ¼ cup Worcestershire sauce
- 1 tablespoon white sugar
- ¼ cup white vinegar
- 1 pinch ground cloves

- 1 quart mayonnaise
- ¾ cup sweet pickle relish
- ½ cup chopped black olives
- ½ cup diced red bell pepper

Directions:

1. Place eggs in a saucepan and cover with cold water. Bring water to a boil and immediately remove from heat. Cover and let eggs stand in hot water for 10 to 12 minutes. Remove from hot water, cool, peel, and chop.
2. In a medium bowl, whisk together chopped eggs, Worcestershire sauce, sugar, vinegar, cloves, mayonnaise, relish, olives, and red pepper until evenly combined.
3. Chill and serve spooned over fresh greens. Store in the refrigerator.

Nutritional Value (Amount per Serving):

Calories: 52; Fat: 2.63; Carb: 5.53; Protein: 1.91

Healthy Tartar Sauce

Prep Time: 10 Minutes   Cook Time: 10 Minutes   Serves: 10

Ingredients:

- 1 egg yolk (Optional)
- 1 cup fat-free mayonnaise

- 2 tablespoons diced cucumber
- ½ lemon, juiced

- 1 tablespoon diced onion
- 1 ½ teaspoons white vinegar
- 1 teaspoon mustard
- 1 small garlic clove, pressed

Directions:

1. Beat egg yolk and mayonnaise together in a bowl; stir cucumber, lemon juice, onion, vinegar, mustard, and garlic into the mayonnaise mixture.
2. Cover bowl with plastic wrap and refrigerate at least 1 hour.

Nutritional Value (Amount per Serving):

Calories: 34; Fat: 0.54; Carb: 6.44; Protein: 1.32

Homemade Tomato Sauce

Prep Time: 30 Minutes   Cook Time: 4 Hours 10 Minutes   Serves: 6

Ingredients:

- 10 ripe tomatoes
- 2 tablespoons butter
- 2 tablespoons olive oil
- 2 small carrots, chopped
- 1 onion, chopped
- 1 small green bell pepper, chopped
- 4 cloves garlic, minced
- ¼ cup Burgundy wine
- ¼ cup chopped fresh basil
- ¼ teaspoon Italian seasoning
- 2 stalks celery
- 1 bay leaf
- 2 tablespoons tomato paste

Directions:

1. Bring a large pot of water to a boil. Prepare a large bowl of ice water.
2. Plunge whole tomatoes in boiling water until skin starts to peel, about 1 minute. Remove with a slotted spoon and place in ice bath. Let rest until cool enough to handle.
3. Remove peels, squeeze out seeds and chop 8 tomatoes.
4. Puree tomatoes in a blender or food processor until smooth. Chop remaining 2 tomatoes and set aside.
5. Heat butter and oil in a large pot or Dutch oven over medium heat. Add carrots, onion, bell pepper, and garlic; cook and stir until onion softens, about 5 minutes.
6. Pour in pureed tomatoes, then stir in chopped tomatoes, wine, basil, and Italian seasoning. Place celery stalks and bay leaf in the pot and bring to a boil. Reduce heat to low, cover, and simmer for 2 hours.
7. Stir in tomato paste; simmer for an additional 2 hours. Discard celery and bay leaf and serve.

Nutritional Value (Amount per Serving):

Calories: 138; Fat: 8.88; Carb: 14.11; Protein: 2.84

Spinach Basil Pesto

Prep Time: 20 Minutes   Cook Time: 20 Minutes   Serves: 24

- 1 ½ cups baby spinach leaves
- ¾ cup fresh basil leaves
- ½ cup toasted pine nuts
- ½ cup grated Parmesan cheese
- ½ cup extra-virgin olive oil, divided
- 4 cloves garlic, peeled and quartered
- 1 tablespoon fresh lemon juice
- ¾ teaspoon kosher salt
- ½ teaspoon lemon zest
- ½ teaspoon freshly ground black pepper

1. Place spinach, basil, pine nuts, Parmesan cheese, 2 tablespoons olive oil, garlic, lemon juice, salt, lemon zest, and pepper into a food processor; blend until nearly smooth, scraping the sides of the bowl with a spatula as necessary.
2. Drizzle remaining olive oil into the mixture while processing until smooth.

Calories: 48; Fat: 4.58; Carb: 0.94; Protein: 1.24

Garlic Scape Pesto

Prep Time: 10 Minutes   Cook Time: 10 Minutes   Serves: 28

- 1 pound garlic scapes, cut into 2-inch pieces
- 1 ¼ cups grated Parmesan cheese
- 1 cup olive oil
- 1 tablespoon lemon juice
- ground black pepper to taste

1. Blend garlic scapes, Parmesan cheese, olive oil, lemon juice, and pepper together in a food processor until smooth.

Calories: 112; Fat: 9.04; Carb: 6.17; Protein: 2.33

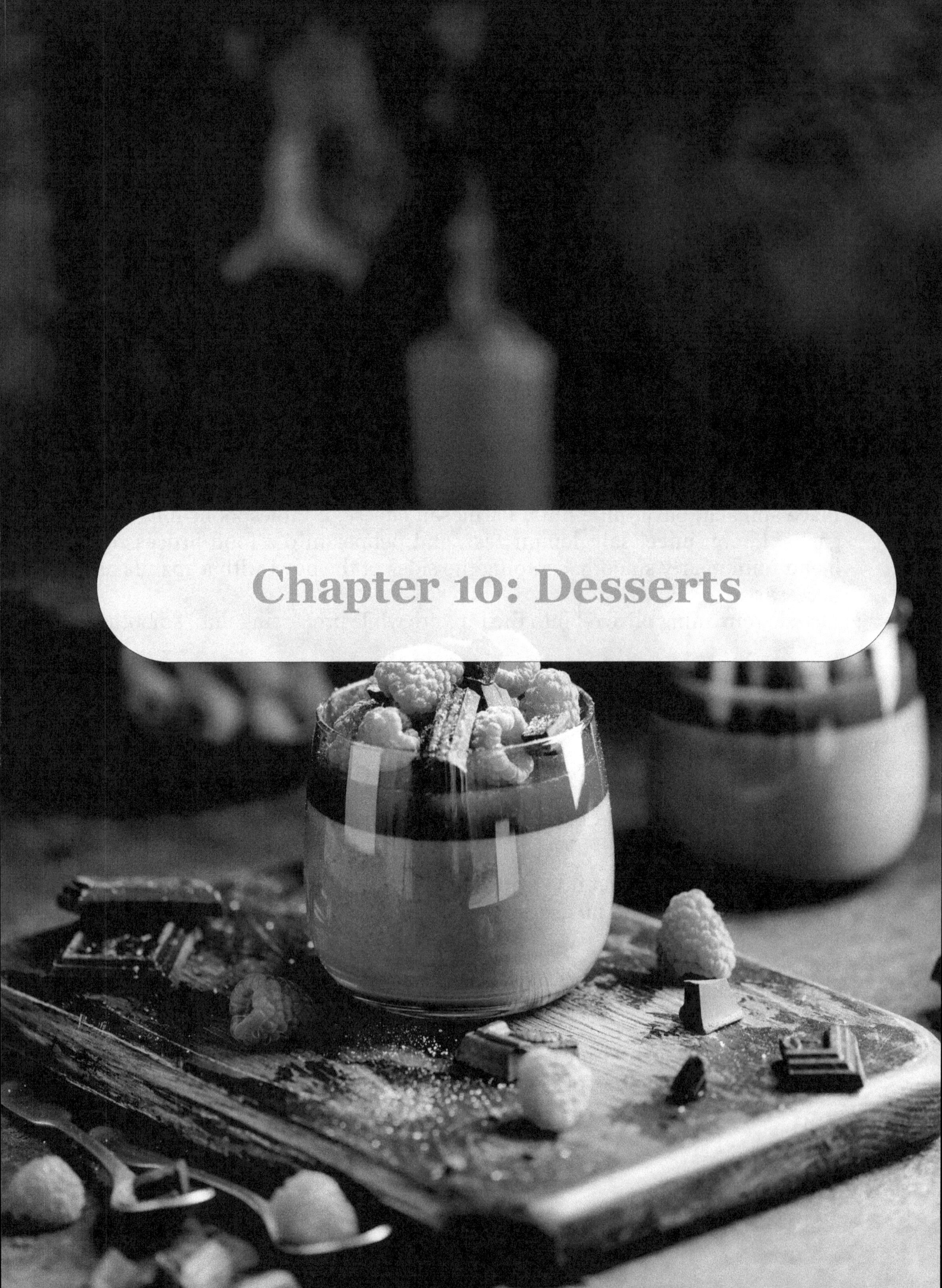

Chapter 10: Desserts

Fruity Fun Skewers

Prep Time: 15 Minutes   Cook Time: 15 Minutes   Serves:5

Ingredients:

- 5 large strawberries, halved
- ¼ cantaloupe, cut into balls or cubes
- 2 bananas, peeled and cut into chunks
- 1 medium apple, cut into chunks
- 20 skewers

Directions:

1. Thread strawberries, cantaloupe, banana, and apple pieces alternately onto skewers, placing at least 2 pieces of fruit on each skewer. Arrange skewers decoratively on a serving platter.
2. Refrigerate for up to 1 day.

Nutritional Value (Amount per Serving):

Calories: 163; Fat: 0.84; Carb: 41.78; Protein: 1.78

Cherry Squares

Prep Time: 20 Minutes   Cook Time: 55 Minutes   Serves:36

Ingredients:

- 1 ¼ cups all-purpose flour
- ⅓ cup packed brown sugar
- ½ cup butter or margarine
- 2 large eggs
- 1 ¼ cups packed brown sugar
- 1 tablespoon all-purpose flour
- ½ teaspoon baking powder
- ⅛ teaspoon salt
- 1 cup flaked coconut
- ½ cup chopped walnuts
- ½ cup maraschino cherries, chopped
- 1 cup confectioners' sugar
- 2 tablespoons butter
- ½ teaspoon vanilla extract
- 1 tablespoon water

Directions:

1. Preheat the oven to 350 degrees F.
2. Prepare the cookie crust: Stir together flour and brown sugar in a medium bowl. Rub in butter using your hands or a pastry blender. Press into an ungreased 9-inch square pan.
3. Bake in the preheated oven until lightly browned at the edges, about 15 minutes. Set aside.
4. Make the cookie filling: Beat eggs in a medium bowl until light. Mix together brown sugar, flour, baking powder, and salt; stir into eggs. Mix in coconut, walnuts, and cherries; spread the batter evenly over the baked crust.

5. Return to the oven and bake until brown, about 25 minutes. Set aside to cool.
6. Make the frosting: Mix confectioners' sugar, butter, water, and vanilla in a small bowl until smooth. Add more liquid if necessary to make a more spreadable mixture. Spread over cooled bars before cutting into squares.
7. Wrap airtight and refrigerate for up to 2 days or freeze for up to 3 months.

Nutritional Value (Amount per Serving):

Calories: 104; Fat: 4.18; Carb: 16.24; Protein: 0.88

Black Raspberry Cobbler

Prep Time: 10 Minutes   Cook Time: 30 Minutes   Serves:8

Ingredients:

- ½ cup melted butter
- 1 ¼ cups white sugar
- 1 cup all-purpose flour
- ¾ cup milk
- 1 ½ teaspoons baking powder
- 2 ½ cups black raspberries

Directions:

1. Preheat the oven to 350 degrees F.
2. Pour melted butter into an 11x7-inch baking dish.
3. Mix 1 cup sugar, flour, milk, and baking powder together in a bowl. Pour on top of melted butter in the baking dish, making sure not to stir. Place black raspberries on top of mixture, making sure not to stir. Top with remaining 1/4 cup sugar.
4. Bake in the preheated oven until crust is browned and set, 30 to 40 minutes.
5. Wrap airtight and refrigerate for up to 2 days.

Nutritional Value (Amount per Serving):

Calories: 315; Fat: 18.53; Carb: 36.09; Protein: 4.02

Summer Fresh Raspberry Pie

Prep Time: 10 Minutes   Cook Time: 1 Hour 25 Minutes   Serves:8

Ingredients:

- 4 cups fresh raspberries, divided
- ½ cup water
- 2 tablespoons cornstarch
- ¼ cup cold water
- ½ cup white sugar
- 1 tablespoon lemon juice

- 1 (9 inch) ready-to-use refrigerated pie crust
- 1 cup whipped cream for garnish
- 1 teaspoon lemon zest for garnish

Directions:

1. Cook 1 cup raspberries and 1/2 cup water in a small saucepan over medium heat, stirring occasionally, until raspberries soften, about 5 minutes. Strain mixture into a bowl through a fine mesh sieve; discard seeds. Return mashed berries to the saucepan.
2. Stir cornstarch into 1/4 cup cold water in a bowl until dissolved. Pour mixture into the saucepan and mix with mashed berries. Stir in sugar. Heat over medium heat, stirring constantly, until thickened, about 5 minutes. Stir in lemon juice. Let cool to room temperature, 15 to 25 minutes.
3. Pour remaining 3 cups raspberries into pie crust. Pour raspberry sauce over top and refrigerate until set, about 1 hour.
4. Garnish slices with whipped cream and lemon zest.
5. Wrap airtight and refrigerate for up to 2 days.

Nutritional Value (Amount per Serving):

Calories: 253; Fat: 9.42; Carb: 42.24; Protein: 2.37

Grandma's Raspberry Bars

Prep Time: 20 Minutes   Cook Time: 30 Minutes   Serves:24

Ingredients:

- ¾ cup butter, softened
- ½ cup white sugar
- ½ cup brown sugar
- 1 ½ cups all-purpose flour
- 1 teaspoon baking powder
- ¼ teaspoon salt
- ¾ cup raspberry jam
- 1 ½ cups rolled oats
- ½ cup chopped walnuts

Directions:

1. Preheat oven to 350 degrees F. Grease a 9x13 inch baking dish.
2. In a medium bowl combine butter, white sugar, brown sugar, flour, baking powder and salt; mix well. Spread 2/3 of mixture into prepared pan.
3. Spread jam over mixture.
4. Combine remaining mixture with oats and walnuts; sprinkle over jam layer.
5. Bake in preheated oven for 30 minutes.
6. Store in refrigerator for up to 4 days.

Nutritional Value (Amount per Serving):

Calories: 139; Fat: 8.14; Carb: 17.07; Protein: 2.33

Vanilla Frozen Yogurt

Prep Time: 5 Minutes   Cook Time: 3 Hours 15Minutes   Serves: 6

Ingredients:

- 3 cups nonfat Greek yogurt
- ⅔ cup white sugar
- 1 teaspoon vanilla extract

Directions:

1. Stir together yogurt, sugar, and vanilla in a bowl until sugar is dissolved. Cover and refrigerate for 1 hour.
2. Pour chilled mixture into an ice cream maker and freeze according to the manufacturer's directions until it reaches "soft-serve" consistency.
3. Transfer to a 1- or 2-quart plastic container with a lid; cover surface with plastic wrap and seal.
4. Allow frozen yogurt to ripen in the freezer for at least 2 hours or overnight.

Nutritional Value (Amount per Serving):

Calories: 68; Fat: 4.41; Carb: 3.92; Protein: 3.53

Banana Protein Muffins

Prep Time: 10 Minutes   Cook Time: 35 Minutes   Serves:12

Ingredients:

- 1 ½ cups white whole-wheat flour
- 1 teaspoon baking powder
- 1 teaspoon ground cinnamon
- ¾ teaspoon baking soda
- ½ teaspoon salt
- ⅓ cup plain whole-milk Greek yogurt
- ⅓ cup creamy natural peanut butter, well stirred
- 2 large eggs
- 1 cup mashed banana (from 2 very ripe bananas)
- ½ cup packed light brown sugar
- ⅓ cup granulated sugar
- 1 teaspoon vanilla extract
- ¾ cup chopped walnuts, toasted

Directions:

1. Preheat oven to 350°F. Line a 12-cup muffin tin with paper liners. Whisk flour, baking powder, cinnamon, baking soda and salt together in a medium bowl. Set aside.
2. Whisk yogurt and peanut butter together in a large bowl until smooth.

Add eggs, banana, brown sugar, granulated sugar and vanilla; whisk to combine. Fold the flour mixture into the banana mixture until the flour is mostly incorporated.

3. Spoon the batter evenly into the prepared muffin cups (3 heaping tablespoons each); sprinkle evenly with walnuts. Bake until a wooden pick inserted in the centers comes out clean, 18 to 22 minutes. Remove from oven; let cool for 5 minutes. Serve warm or let cool completely, about 30 minutes.
4. Wrap airtight and refrigerate for up to 2 days or freeze for up to 3 months.

Nutritional Value (Amount per Serving):

Calories: 192; Fat: 8.57; Carb: 25.34; Protein: 5.23

Carolyn's Oh-So-Easy Cherry Cobbler

Prep Time: 10 Minutes   Cook Time: 25 Minutes   Serves: 6

Ingredients:

- 1 (15 ounce) can pitted tart red cherries, drained with liquid reserved
- ½ cup sugar
- 1 cup buttermilk baking mix
- ½ cup sugar
- ½ cup milk

Directions:

1. Preheat oven to 350 degrees F. Prepare a 9x9-inch baking dish with cooking spray.
2. Stir the liquid from the cherries and 1/2 cup sugar together in a small glass bowl; heat in the microwave until the sugar is dissolved, 1 to 2 minutes. Set aside.
3. Stir the baking mix, 1/2 cup sugar, and milk together in a separate small bowl; mix until you get a moist batter. Spread the mixture in an even layer in the bottom of the prepared baking dish. Spread the cherries evenly over the batter. Slowly pour the cherry juice over the cherries.
4. Bake in the preheated oven until lightly browned, 25 to 30 minutes. Refrigerate for up to 2 days.

Nutritional Value (Amount per Serving):

Calories: 119; Fat: 1.32; Carb: 26.28; Protein: 1.54

Tart Cherry Cobbler

Prep Time: 20 Minutes   Cook Time: 1 Hour 45 Minutes   Serves: 12

Ingredients:

- 5 (14.5 ounce) cans tart pitted cherries packed in water, drained
- 1 cup brown sugar

- ½ cup white sugar
- 3 tablespoons quick-cooking tapioca
- ½ teaspoon almond extract
- ¼ teaspoon cinnamon
- 1 pinch salt
- 1 tablespoon butter, diced
- 1 recipe pastry for double-crust pie
- 2 tablespoons milk

Directions:

1. Preheat oven to 400 degrees F.
2. In a large bowl, gently stir the cherries, brown sugar, and white sugar until all the sugar has dissolved. Mix in the tapioca, almond extract, cinnamon, and salt. Let stand 15 minutes. Pour into a 9x13 inch baking dish, and dot with butter.
3. Roll our pie pastry into a rectangle slightly larger than the baking dish, and place over the cherries. Tuck in corners, and make several slits in the dough. Brush with milk.
4. Bake 45 minutes in the preheated oven, until crust is lightly browned and filling is bubbly. Cool 1 hour before serving.
5. Refrigerate for up to 2 days.

Nutritional Value (Amount per Serving):

Calories: 198; Fat: 7.9; Carb: 31.5; Protein: 1.59

Sweet and Silky Strawberry Sorbet

Prep Time: 15 Minutes   Cook Time: 2 Hours 5 Minutes   Serves: 4

Ingredients:

- 1 pound ripe strawberries, hulled and chopped
- ½ cup white sugar
- 1 pinch salt
- 1 ½ teaspoons cornstarch
- 1 ½ teaspoons cold water
- 3 tablespoons lemon juice

Directions:

1. Place berries in the bowl of a food processor and purée until smooth. Pour mixture into a large saucepan over medium heat. Add sugar and salt; stir until dissolved and bring to a simmer.
2. Whisk together cornstarch and cold water in a small bowl; stir into simmering berry mixture. Remove the saucepan from heat, stir in lemon juice, and allow to cool slightly. Refrigerate berry mixture until cold, about 2 hours.
3. Freeze in an ice cream maker according to manufacturer's instructions. Freeze for up to 2 days.

Calories: 98; Fat: 5.18; Carb: 13.56; Protein: 1.52

Fresh Fig Cake

Prep Time: 40 Minutes   Cook Time: 30 Minutes   Serves: 8

Ingredients:

- ¼ cup butter, softened
- 1 cup white sugar
- 1 egg
- 2 cups all-purpose flour
- ½ teaspoon salt
- 2 teaspoons baking powder
- 1 cup fat-free evaporated milk
- 1 teaspoon vanilla extract
- ¼ teaspoon almond extract
- 1 cup chopped fresh figs
- 2 cups chopped fresh figs
- ¼ cup packed brown sugar
- ¼ cup water
- 1 tablespoon lemon juice

Directions:

1. Preheat oven to 350 degrees F. Spray two 8-inch round cake pans with vegetable oil spray.
2. In a medium bowl, sift together flour, salt and baking powder. Set aside.
3. In a large mixing bowl, cream butter with the sugar until fluffy. Add egg and beat well. Add flour mixture alternately with the evaporated milk. Fold in vanilla and almond extracts and 1 cup chopped figs.
4. Divide into two prepared 8-inch round cake pans. Bake in preheated oven until cake springs back when lightly touched with a fingertip and a toothpick inserted into the center comes out clean, 25 to 30 minutes. Cool cake layers on wire rack.
5. To make the filling: In a saucepan, combine 2 cups chopped figs, brown sugar, water and lemon juice. Bring to a boil. Reduce heat to a simmer and cook until thickened, about 20 minutes. Spread thinly between cooled cake layers and on top.
6. Store in the refrigerator for up to 3 days.

Nutritional Value (Amount per Serving):

Calories: 416; Fat: 12.69; Carb: 71.85; Protein: 8.05

Granola & Yogurt Breakfast Popsicles

Prep Time: 20 Minutes   Cook Time: 8 Hours   Serves: 6

Ingredients:

- 1 ¼ cups low-fat plain yogurt
- 1 ½ cups chopped fresh berries (strawberries, blueberries, raspberries and/

or blackberries)
- 4 teaspoons pure maple syrup, divided
- 1 teaspoon vanilla extract
- 6 tablespoons granola, large chunks crumbled

Directions:

1. Stir yogurt, berries, 2 teaspoons maple syrup and vanilla together in a medium bowl. Divide among six 3-ounce popsicle molds. Stir granola and the remaining 2 teaspoons maple syrup together in a small bowl. Top each popsicle with 1 tablespoon of the granola mixture. Insert popsicle sticks and freeze overnight.
2. Store popsicles in the freezer for up to 1 week.

Nutritional Value (Amount per Serving):

Calories: 138; Fat: 5.75; Carb: 17.32; Protein: 3.98

Chia Seed Pudding for dessert

Prep Time: 15 Minutes   Cook Time: 8 Hours   Serves: 4-5

Ingredients:

- 2 cups light coconut milk or homemade almond milk
- 6 tablespoons chia seeds
- 1 tablespoon maple syrup
- ¼ teaspoon cinnamon
- ⅛ teaspoon sea salt

Directions:

1. In a lidded 3- to 4-cup jar, combine the milk, chia seeds, maple syrup, cinnamon, and salt. Cover and shake to combine. Chill for a few hours, then give it a good stir to loosen any clumps. Continue chilling for 12 to 18 hours for the pudding to set.

Nutritional Value (Amount per Serving):

Calories: 362; Fat: 33.22; Carb: 16.46; Protein: 5.24

APPENDIX RECIPE INDEX